PRAISE FOR THE PINTEREST DIET

"Mitzi is a Pinterest POWERHOUSE! I love the concrete strategies she lays out in this book, delivered with her contagious enthusiasm. Mitzi shows you how to use this unique social media platform to gather all the resources, inspiration, and support you need to lose weight and transform your life."

—Cynthia Sass, MPH, RD, author of the New York Times bestseller *S.A.S.S!
Yourself Slim*, nutritionist for *HEALTH* magazine.

"In Mitzi's groundbreaking work, The Pinterest Diet, she combines her powerful Pinterest know-how with her skills as a dietitian, personal trainer, and social media expert to create an innovative program for using social media to help you lose weight and transform your life. This book is BRILLIANT!"

—Cheryl Forberg, RD, James Beard award-winning chef and nutritionist for NBC's *The Biggest Loser*

"Mitzi has created an ingeniously SIMPLE, FUN new approach to LOSING WEIGHT—permanently. Readers will love The Pinterest Diet's tasty, satisfying recipes and its calorie-torching workouts. And they'll be amazed at the results they get! Mitzi's social media expertise and her ability to translate complex topics into bite-size morsels make this book a must-have!"

—Christopher R. Mohr, PhD, RD, Owner of Mohr Results, Inc., sports nutritionist for the Cincinnati Bengals

"Mitzi's program harnesses the power of Pinterest to help you lose weight, find inspiration, and eat delicious foods for every meal. The Pinterest Diet shows you how to use your favorite digital-age tool in a way that works for YOU. This book will transform your life!"

—Kate Geagan, RD, author of *Go Green Get Lean*

The
PINTEREST
DIET

How to
Pin Your
Way Thin

Mitzi Dulan, RD America's Nutrition Expert®
and #1 Nutritionist on Pinterest

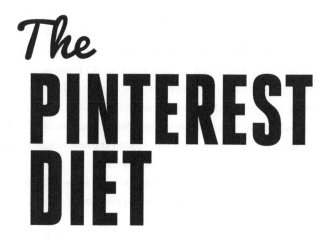

The
PINTEREST
DIET

This book is intended as a reference only, not a medical manual. The information provided in it is designed to help you make informed decisions about your health. In no way is it intended as a substitute for any treatment prescribed by your physician. If you feel that you might have a medical problem, we highly encourage you to seek medical attention. All forms of exercise pose inherent risks. We advise readers to take full responsibility for their safety and know their limits.

The exercise and dietary regimens in this book are not intended as a substitute for any dietary regimen or exercise routine that may have been prescribed by your doctor. This book is meant to supplement, not replace proper exercise training. As with any new weight-loss plan or exercise program, you should get your doctor's approval before starting.

The author and publisher specifically disclaim all responsibility for any liability or loss incurred as a consequence, directly or indirectly, of the use and application of any of the contents of this book.

Mention of specific companies and organizations in this book does not imply endorsement by the author or publisher, nor does mention of specific companies and organizations imply that they endorse this book, its author, or publisher.

This book is not meant to provide legal advice, and the author and publisher do not provide legal services. If legal advice is required, the legal services of a competent legal professional should be sought.

The author does have spokesperson relationships with some brands included in this book.

Internet addresses given in this book were accurate at the time it went to press.

© 2013 by Mitzi Dulan

The Library of Congress Cataloging-in-Publication Data

Dulan, Mitzi.

The Pinterest Diet : How To Pin Your Way Thin / By Mitzi Dulan.

ISBN: 978-0-9897239-4-7

Photographs: Jeff Nicholson, Mark Lea

Cover Design: Georgia Morrissey

To My Mom
Thanks For Loving Me So Much!
I Miss You.

TABLE OF CONTENTS

ACKNOWLEDGEMENTS

To my husband, Antoine. Thanks for always being a team player in our life. Thanks for putting up with me and with all of my recipe testing in our kitchen. Thanks to my daughters, Josie and Jasmine. My life is truly full because of both of you. I'm grateful that you were both always ready and willing to taste Mommy's newest recipes for this book.

Thank you to my incredible book doctor and editor, Kathy Passero, for sharing your amazing talent on a tight timeline.

Julie May, my manager. I feel so lucky and honored to work with such a caring and smart person. Thanks for all your guidance.

Kate Geagan, my good friend and colleague. Thank you so much for the many years of friendship and wisdom you have shared with me.

Thanks to my wonderful mastermind group and colleagues who have supported me and have all become my dear friends: Cynthia Sass, Cheryl Forberg, Chris Mohr, Robin Plotkin, Lisa Sutherland, Cindy Heroux, Kristen Carlucci, and Shelly Marie Redmond.

My great virtual interns, who have been so fun to work with: Morgan Hoover, Faith Doan, Katie Hipwell, and Iakhabue Akhabue.

To my fabulous group of girlfriends who first told me about Pinterest (Jenny Jehlik and Heidi Cassaday) and many others who were so understanding while I was writing this book and had to say no to some fun get-togethers: Amanda Koffman, Theresa Nuss, Tamara Hutcheson, Linda Mills, Patti Puricelli, Tina Miller, and Betsy Berkley. I truly appreciate all the support you have given me. I am very blessed to be surrounded with such a great group of girlfriends.

Thanks to all my amazing clients.

Thanks to Art Allen for your generosity.

Thanks to the rest of my family for all your support.

—Mitzi Dulan

CHAPTER 1:

LET'S DO THIS!

"You don't have to be great to start, but you have to start to be great." —Anonymous

Want To Pin Your Way Thin In 30 Days?

About 50 million Americans go on a diet every year. If you're reading this book, chances are you're one of them. And, if so, you know how tough it can be. That's because most diets are all about what I call the "three Ds." Discipline. Denial. And deprivation.

Forget the three Ds! In this book, I'm going to teach you an amazingly simple, fun new way to shape up, shed unwanted pounds, and develop healthy eating habits you can live with happily for the rest of your life—all using the incredible power of Pinterest.

Believe it or not, Pinterest.com can change your life.

If you've never checked it out, Pinterest is a mammoth social media scrapbook, loaded with breathtaking colorful photos and intriguing articles pinned by its millions of users to virtual pin boards that are grouped by interest so they're well-organized and super easy to find. It's free. It's easy to use. It's a clutter-cutter. And it's a goldmine of inspiration. What's really exciting is that Pinterest's offerings change and expand every day because users are constantly adding new pins.

What makes Pinterest the perfect medium for dieters? To borrow an old cliché, a picture is worth a thousand words. That's especially true when it comes to keeping yourself motivated in trying to lose weight and live healthier. All those gorgeous visual cues make it a cinch to pin your way thin.

Feeling hungry? Just log in and go to your MSF Factor Foods Board, to find easy-to-make satisfying snacks.

Bored with your gym routine? Glance at your Workout Plans Board to find a few quick ways to spice it up.

Feel like giving up? Refocus with a look at your Daily Inspiration Board, featuring the perfect little black dress you plan to buy when you reach your goal.

"Every accomplishment starts with the decision to try."
—Anonymous

Pin 10! 10 Minutes Is All It Takes

Following the simple how-to's in this book, you can create your own unique collection of Pinterest boards, tailored to your goals, your preferences, and your passions. You'll fill them with the images and information that inspire you most, adding more and updating them as you work toward your goal. All you need is 10 minutes a day to devote to pinning. (You'll see "Pin 10" tips throughout the book to remind you of this simple, essential strategy.)

I'll walk you through every step and give you lots of great places where you can find pins. I encourage you to repin from my own boards (I'll give you a list of board titles). I'll also give you a list of some of my favorite trustworthy health and fitness sources to find pins, such as Shape.com. (I've included a handy list of these in chapter three.) Finally, don't be afraid to have fun mixing in your own photos, recipes, and inspiring quotes.

Along the way, you'll discover how addictively enjoyable Pinterest can be. (I'm guessing you'll soon discover that 10 minutes a day isn't nearly enough to devote to pinning!) To me, logging onto Pinterest is like going to the bookstore and having all your favorite magazines in front of you, going to the grocery store and having all your favorite foods in front of you, and hearing all the words you need to stay motivated—all in one convenient spot.

All those beautiful, colorful visual cues will help to build your awareness of delicious food and fitness options. They'll boost your morale when it gets low. Instead of the dreaded "three Ds" that have made so many dieters despair, your Pinterest boards will buoy your spirits and energize you. Best of all, Pinterest's streamlined format keeps everything you need organized and easy to access at a glance 24-7 on your laptop, desktop, or handheld mobile device. You'll even have a collection of delicious, diet-approved recipes on hand when you're at the grocery store. Just check your smartphone to find out which ingredients to buy.

My Pinterest Home Page

"The journey of a thousand miles begins with one step."
—Lao Tzu

Mitzi's Story: How I Discovered Pinterest

I earned my degrees and launched my career as a nutritionist long before Pinterest existed. Today, I'm grateful to have nearly 3.8 million Pinterest followers. I love reading all their comments about my pins and repins.

In addition to my millions of Pinterest followers, I work one-on-one with clients from all walks of life—from young moms with growing families to professional athletes in my role as the team nutritionist for the Kansas City Royals Baseball Team and the former longtime team nutritionist for the Kansas City Chiefs.

The challenge, no matter who I work with, is to develop a diet plan that delivers 100% satisfaction with no deprivation. That means my clients' meals have to be packed with nutrient-rich foods, they have to taste wonderful, and they have to leave the person who eats them feeling completely well fed. I work closely with all my clients, helping them tweak and modify their meal plans to suit their needs. You have to make it fun, interesting, and rewarding or people will give up before they reach their goals.

A few years ago, I would never have imagined that I could do that through an online community. How could I help people reach their goals if I couldn't sit down with them to talk it through? Wouldn't any online diet have to be a cookie-cutter program?

When two of my closest friends first mentioned Pinterest, I dismissed it. I'd never heard of the site and couldn't even understand what they were calling it. To tell the truth, I didn't even take the trouble to check it out. I was writing for other websites as well as magazines, and my schedule was jam-packed as usual.

But then, after an article titled "A Day in My Diet" was posted on Shape. com profiling everything I ate during a 24-hour period in January of 2012, I noticed a "Pin It" button on the article. I checked back a few days later to find that several people had "pinned" it.

Time to take a closer look at Pinterest.

From the moment I joined Pinterest, I was enthralled. I love to look at great food photos and try new recipes. Pinterest turned out to be a garden of culinary delights. So many delicious-looking recipes! I loved trying them. And I quickly found that I could modify them to improve the nutritional value while maintaining the flavor. I started re-pinning other people's recipes, with "Mitzi's Modifications" to make them healthier by using "cleaner" ingredients. (More on clean eating and modifying recipes later.) I created boards for different categories. Before long, hundreds of people starting responding to what they saw on my boards. Soon thousands—and then millions—of people were responding and repinning my pins.

Know The Lingo: Pinterest Terms

Board: A board is where you organize your pins by topic. Boards can be secret or public, and you can invite other people to pin with you on any of your boards.

Follow: When you "follow" someone, their pins show up in your Pinterest home feed. You can follow all of someone's boards or just the ones you like best.

Like: Users can click the "like" button to let the original pinner know they enjoyed their pin. When you "like" an image, it gets added to the Likes section of your Pinterest user profile.

Pin: A pin starts with an image or video you add to Pinterest. You can add a pin from a website using the Pin It "bookmarklet" or upload an image right from your computer. Any pin on Pinterest can be repinned, and all pins link back to their source.

Pinner: A Pinterest user.

Repin: Repinning happens when you pin an image from someone else's Pinterest board to one of your own boards—or when someone else pins an image from one of your boards to one of theirs. The person who first pinned the image still gets credit for it, and the source-link still appears, repinned.

Courtesy of Pinterest.com and Pinterest Guide: The Ultimate Guide to Creative and Money Making Ideas with Pinterest by Maddie Alexander

Getting Started

You can sign up for Pinterest using your Facebook account, your Twitter account, or your email address. If you want more privacy, you're better off using your email address.

1. Go to the Pinterest homepage at Pinterest.com.
2. Click the "Join Pinterest" button.
3. Click on the option you want to use to join. You'll have to log into Facebook to join that way.
4. Choose a user name, type in your email address, and create a password.
5. An "Add Interests" page will appear. Click on the topics that pique your interest, from "recipes" to "exercise."

What an affirmation! When I discovered how many people were enjoying the recipes I had pinned and repinned, it was like having guests at a table that stretched out for miles and miles. Today it's not uncommon for me to get as many as 4,000 repins to a single recipe or meal plan I pin. In fact, I've had more than 55,000 pins of my most popular recipe ever, the *Skinny Strawberry Sangria,* directly from my website! But a recipe board wasn't enough. I've always loved motivational quotes. Often I come across great ones that make me stop and think about what I'm doing. Quotes help me stay focused on my goals. They remind me of what it means to live in a place of gratitude and contentment— and to think about how I can improve myself and make a difference in the world. I believe inspirational quotes are essential for anyone making a real commitment to a healthier lifestyle and to creating a better life. I always want to strive to be the best person I can be, and I've found that quotes help me move in a positive direction.

I also created a Workout Plans Board, which includes recipes and quotes as well as exercises. This has become my most popular board, based on the enthusiastic feedback I get from my many followers.

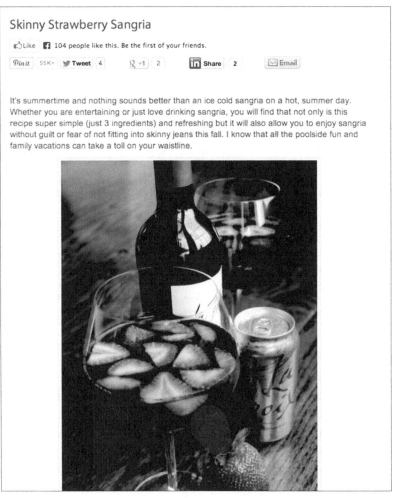

My Skinny Strawberry Sangria Blog With Over 55,000 Pins

Pinterest By The Numbers

- Pinterest was created in 2009 by 27-year-old former Yale student Ben Silbermann
- Pinterest now has 70 million users
- Pinterest is worth $7.7 billion as a company
- 15 percent of adult U.S. Internet users use Pinterest
- 85% of Pinterest users are women
- Women are five times more likely to use Pinterest than men
- Most women using Pinterest are between the ages of 25 and 54
- The average Pinterest user has 2,757 pins, 35 boards, and 355 followers
- When pinners see a "call to action" pin, they're 80% more likely to be engaged or follow through on a project or activity
- The average time spent on Pinterest per visit is 14.2 minutes
- 57% of Pinterest users interact with food-related content—it's the #1 category of content
  Source: Pew Research, Forbes, Techcrunch.com, TheNextWeb.com

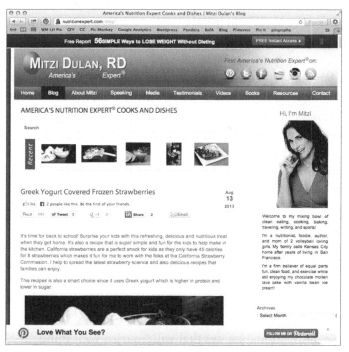

My Blog

"Never give up on a dream just because of the time it will take to accomplish it. The time will pass anyway."
—*Earl Nightingale*

Time To Change Your Life!

What does it all mean? It's proof positive that people really can use Pinterest to improve their lives.

Pinterest puts everything you need to stay on track at your fingertips—from mouthwatering recipes for brightly colored fruit smoothies and gooey black-bean brownies to innovative workouts. You can even fill your boards with inspiring photos of slimming swim fashions for the beach . . . and dreamy tropical destinations where you can envision yourself wearing them.

Seeing inspires us. It motivates us. It energizes us and gives us fresh ideas.

That's why Pinterest works. It's the reason that millions of users, including myself, enjoy it so much and can't wait to log on every day, whether it's for a few quick minutes or to savor it at leisure.

Pinterest has become an important part of my life. It's not just for pleasure, though the site is great fun. These days, I use Pinterest in more ways than I could ever have imagined. Pinterest has become my personal record-keeper, my inspiration guide, my favorite "go-to" cookbook, my news source, and my health and fitness library—all rolled into one. It has broadened my horizons, encouraged me, and literally changed my life.

Now it can do the same for you.

In the following chapters, I'll show you how incredibly easy it is to use Pinterest to achieve lasting weight-loss and better health.

You can . . .

- Discover irresistible recipes that feature your favorite satisfying, nutritious, delicious foods by searching for key ingredients like Greek yogurt or strawberries
- Find great new workouts
- Pinpoint ways to improve your health, your fitness level, and your wellbeing
- Find motivational quotes that will nourish your mind
- Keep yourself on the right track in a way that's fun, fresh, and manageable

- and much more!

"To create a pinboard is to say to the world, Here are the beautiful things that make me who I am-—or who I want to be." —Fast Company, October 2012

Respect Copyrights! I am not providing legal advice, so please seek counsel from a competent attorney if you are in doubt about whether something you want to pin or repin is copyright-free or copyright-protected. To fully understand Pinterest's Copyright Policy, visit: about.pinterest.com/copyright/

Penny-Wise! Two-thirds of all Americans are overweight or obese. As a nation, we spend almost $60 billion a year on diet programs and products, according to recent research. The cost to join Pinterest? It's FREE!

Virtual Fridge: Remember the old dieting trick of putting pictures on your refrigerator? The idea was that you'd see the photo of the bathing suit you desperately wanted to fit into by summer (or the unflattering photo of your backside in too-tight white jeans) and you'd reach for the hummus and carrots instead of the Ben & Jerry's. Think of Pinterest as a fresh, new, 21st-century virtual twist on the tried-and-true notion of using fridge pics for inspiration.

Follow Me!
My boards provide you with thousands of recipes for delicious meals and snacks that meet all the requirements for my Pinterest Diet—approved foods. I'll share more about the foods you should eat later.

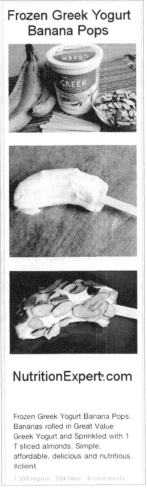

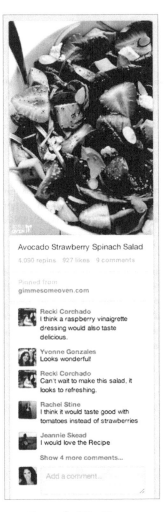

**Frozen Greek Yogurt
Banana Pops**

**Sample Pin From
GimmeSomeOven.com**

You'll also find lots of innovative workouts that I use for my clients and for myself. Pin the plans that you want to try. If you're not sure whether you'll use one, go ahead and pin it. That way, you'll have it on hand when you want to try something new. Experiment with all the exercises that seem interesting to find which work best for you.

On my Daily Inspiration and Workout Plans Boards, you'll find encouraging words, insights, and a little humor to help you stay focused on your weight loss goals.

You can also check out my website (NutritionExpert.com) to find the most up-to-date news about research breakthroughs related to good health, nutrition, and weight-loss.

CHAPTER 2:

5 BOARDS TO TRANSFORM YOUR LIFE

"To change your body, you must change your mind." —Anonymous

Congratulations! You've taken the first step toward pinning your way thin in 30 days. Now that you know the easy basics from chapter one and you've got your own Pinterest account, you're ready to create the five boards that will be your keys to successful weight loss.

Each one is devoted to a different important aspect of healthy living. They include:

1. MSF Factor Foods
2. Workout Plans
3. Daily Inspiration
4. In The Know
5. Favorite Products

You'll fill your boards with the images and information that appeal to you and that apply directly to your goals. I have boards for each of these topics, and I urge you to start creating your own boards by checking out my pins and repinning your favorites. I'll be your chief nutrition and fitness curator. I'll provide you with the most up-to-date nutrition, fitness, and health information. Also, be sure to check out my website (NutritionExpert.com) regularly. I'm always adding new articles, recipes, and workouts—all of which you're free to pin. Reliable health, fitness, and nutrition websites are another great source for pinnable material. To make finding them easy, I've included a list of my favorites in this chapter. Whenever you find something you want to pin, Pinterest automatically creates a link to the website it came from, so you'll be able to find it again easily whenever you need it.

In addition, Pinterest lets you search by key word or click on a list of categories—"Health & Fitness," "Food & Drink," "Quotes," "Humor," and so on—to find images you might want to pin to your boards.

Finally, don't be afraid to take your own snapshots and upload them as pins. Experts estimate that more than 80% of the content on Pinterest is repinned from other users, but if you want to do it yourself, go for it!

Here's a brief guide to creating the boards that will transform your life.

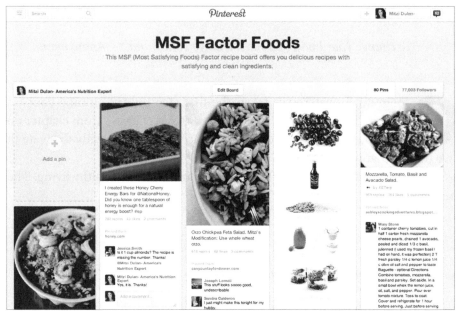

My MSF Factor Foods Board

What to pin:

- Recipes, recipes, and more recipes—for meals, snacks, appetizers, sides, warm and cold beverages, smoothies, salads, sandwiches, soups, stews, spreads, sauces, dips, desserts, and more
- Food charts and lists
- Food and nutrition facts
- Food shopping tips
- Timesaving cooking ideas

#1: MSF Factor Foods Board

One of the best and most unique features of *The Pinterest Diet* is that you'll never feel deprived on it. That's because your diet will be rich in what I call MSF Factor Foods. "MSF" stands for Most Satisfying Foods. You'll find out all about MSFs in chapter four. In short, MSF Factor foods are sources of protein, healthy fats, and/or fiber. They provide you with the long-term satisfaction you need to make a permanent lifestyle change. My recipes also incorporate lots of foods with antioxidant-boosting power to help you stay healthy while you stay satisfied.

Use your MSF Factor Foods Board to guide your food choices. I'll help you along until you gain a strong understanding of what to look for as you scour recipes on Pinterest, scan a restaurant menu, or head to the grocery store. Using my boards as your primary source, you'll fill your own board with recipes for breakfasts, lunches, brunches, dinners, snacks, soups, drinks, and appetizers that feature your favorite healthy MSF foods. If you love spicy dishes, you'll find great ways to add sizzle to salmon on my boards. If you love smoothies, I've got countless mix-in ideas to add nutritious variety.

Whether you've got a craving for a mid-morning snack, you need to get a tasty dinner on the table in 20 minutes, or you're heading to the store to pick up groceries for the week, you can turn to your MSF Factor Foods Board for help. Everything you need will be at your fingertips, easy to find, and visually appealing enough to whet your appetite.

As you create your board, think about your lifestyle. For example, if you've got a busy schedule and hate spending time in the kitchen, pin simple recipes with easy-to-find ingredients. Avoid any that require hours of prep time or include obscure ingredients. Most of the recipes I pin are quick and simple, so please visit my boards to get started! I love to go to the upper left hand corner of my main Pinterest page and type a favorite ingredient like quinoa into the search box. Immediately, Pinterest shows me hundreds of recipes with photos of quinoa recipes. You can even find Quinoa-only boards. Marla Meridith has one with 151 pins. How fun!

Don't try to do all your pinning at once. That can feel overwhelming. Instead, add to your virtual "recipe box" a few times a week. Build it slowly— and take your time trying the dishes you've collected.

As the seasons change, liven up your board with tasty treats that feature your favorite fruits and veggies when they're ripest. You might pin a recipe for frozen watermelon lemonade in the summer and one for baked apples with cinnamon in the fall, for instance. Magazines often feature pinnable seasonal recipes on their websites, which are excellent sources of content for your board.

Remember, too, that Pinterest is designed to be dynamic. Don't be afraid to delete a recipe if it looked delicious, but tasted lackluster.

"Pin It" Bookmarklet

This is a must-have tool on *The Pinterest Diet*. Pinterest offers a "Pin It" bookmarklet button to add to your bookmarks bar on your computer allowing you to create one-click pinning from any website or blog. Let's say, for example, you are reading an article about 8 new ways to incorporate kale into your diet, you can simply click your "Pin It" button, then choose the board you want to pin it to and it's that easy. Now you have easy access to the article anytime you want to refer to it. Download it on Pinterest at: About.Pinterest.com/Goodies/

2: Workout Plans Board

Here's where you'll pin ideas for great workout plans that you find on my Pinterest boards and other trusted sources. You'll also pin exercise-related tidbits, like a list of Top 10 Workout Songs. Pinterest is loaded with step-by-step photos of exercises, charts and diagrams, even videos contributed by certified personal trainers, exercise enthusiasts, and fellow wannabe shape-uppers.

If you're bored with your fitness routine, using your Workout Plans Board is the perfect way to inject new life into it. I've already pinned hundreds of great workouts to my Workout Plans Board, so the easiest way to get started is to go to my board and repin away! Then, take your iPhone with you to the gym, log onto Pinterest, and consult your Workout Plans Board to find out how to spice up your gym time with those new glute, ab, Tabata, or CrossFit workouts you pinned. Too short on time to hit the gym? Not a problem. I have some killer 12-minute workouts that can be done anywhere—in your bedroom, living room, driveway, you name it. More good news: *The Pinterest Diet* Workout: A 30-Day Exercise Plan in chapter 11 maps out an easy-to-follow fitness program for the whole month ahead.

Exercise is an indispensable part of every successful weight-loss program. It's vital to living a healthy lifestyle. If you haven't hit upon an activity you enjoy enough to make it stick as part of your weekly routine, Pinterest can help. Think about your hobbies, your favorite times of day, the seasons when you like to be outdoors, and so on. Do searches to see what ideas turn up. Maybe it's a sunrise yoga routine if you're a morning person. Perhaps it's a pool workout that feels more like play, if you love the water but are bored stiff with swimming laps.

As with your MSF Factor Foods Board, have fun with your Workout Plans Board. Expand it, update it, change it based on what's working best for you. Don't forget to visit my Workout Plans Board daily to see the latest workouts I'm pinning or repinning!

I've created this book to work seamlessly with Pinterest. Using the two together, you'll find it remarkably easy to achieve the goals you've dreamed about.

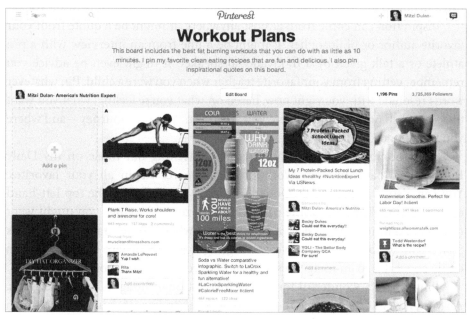

My Workout Plans Board

What to pin:
- Daily or weekly workout plans
- A great workout routine you find on a health magazine's website

- Photographic how-to's and videos of interesting new exercises
- Ab workouts, arm workouts, butt workouts, etc.
- Stretching photos
- Yoga sequences with photos
- Workout music playlists

3: Daily Inspiration Board

This is one of my all-time favorites. I add to my Daily Inspiration Board almost every day, filling it with words that boost my spirits, make me laugh, make me grateful for the little things, and help me keep it all in perspective. Any life-changing journey involves mental and spiritual reflection—especially the journey to health, fitness, and the dream weight that's been eluding you.

Inspiration can come from almost anywhere. It might be a quote from your favorite author or philosopher. It might be a line from an interview with a pro athlete or a talk given by a motivational speaker. It might even be advice you remember getting from your favorite teacher when you were a child. Pin whatever words resonate with you right now, based on what you're feeling, what you want to accomplish or overcome, where you are in your personal journey—and where you want to go.

Start looking for inspirational pins by checking out those on my Daily Inspiration Board and my Workout Plans Board. Repin all your favorites. You can also type the word "Quotes" into the search bar in the top left-hand corner of your Pinterest home page to find dozens of sayings you might want to repin. Another Pinterest tool I love to use when I find a fabulous quote is ShareAsImage.com. It allows you to highlight text anywhere on the web and easily convert it to an image to share on Pinterest, Facebook, or Twitter.

Pinterest is a wonderful forum for inspirational thoughts and reflections. All you have to do is choose the ones that speak to you. If you can't find them on Pinterest or online, upload them yourself.

More than any other, this board will help you through tough times and setbacks. If you're discouraged because you didn't reach your weight loss goal for the month or because in a moment of weakness you downed a heaping helping of double-chocolate fudge cake, turn to your Daily Inspiration Board. It will reassure you, remind you of your accomplishments, set you back on the path to better health, and propel you forward toward your goals.

Your Daily Inspiration Board is also the place to pin inspiring photos. Pin photos of your dream body to keep you focused on your goal. Pin a picture of the white sundress you plan to buy when you reach it. Then add an image of a gorgeous Caribbean island where you can envision yourself wearing it with confidence when you reach your goal. Maybe you'll even decide to reward your hard work with a vacation there!

One of my favorite boards to follow is Helen Hirst's Diet Inspiration Board. Check it out: Pinterest.com/HelenHirst/Diet-Inspiration/

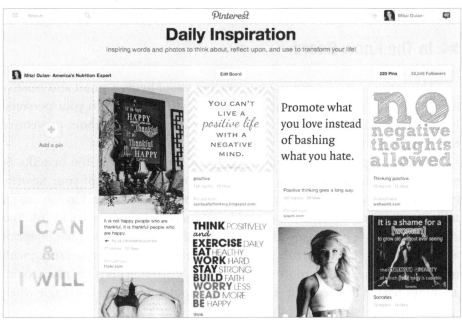

My Daily Inspiration Board

What to pin:
- Quotes from your favorite writers, humorists, world leaders, historical figures, and role models
- Words of encouragement about overcoming obstacles, enjoying life, thinking positive, being in the moment, accepting yourself, dreaming, striving, perseverance, success, and whatever else speaks to you
- Photos of people with the body type you're striving to get

- Pictures of great vacation spots that you'd like to visit as a reward to yourself for transforming your life
- Great clothes and accessories you love to envision yourself wearing when you reach your weight and fitness goals
- Photos of inspiring workout settings you could use (the beach, the park, sunset, etc.)

"Goals are dreams with deadlines."
—Anonymous

#4: In The Know Board

This is the board for general information about living a smart and healthy lifestyle. It's the spot to pin anything and everything related to your personal health, from stress-relief tips to lists of super foods to news about preventive medicine breakthroughs.

It's also a good place to pin images that remind you of the benefits of good health. For example, you might want to include some of your favorite types of active recreation, like cycling along the boardwalk next to the beach, taking a woodland hike with your kids, or gardening in your backyard. You can also showcase other aspects of a healthy lifestyle, like a soothing image of a cozy bedroom conducive to a good night's sleep if you've been wrestling with insomnia or a meditation room if you need to de-stress. This is the place to pin all things related to sleep. (I'll tell you more about it, but sleep is a biggie when it comes to pinning your way thin!)

If you have any specific health concerns, such as high blood pressure or a family history of diabetes, this is the board for prevention tips, reports about new research, and anything else that will help you cope effectively with potential health challenges.

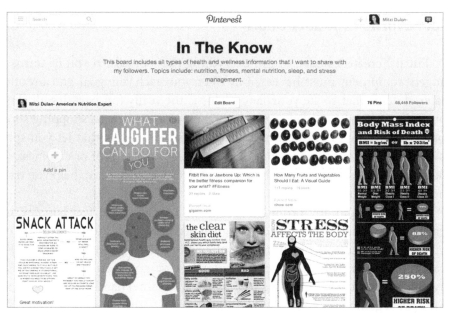

My In The Know Board

What to pin:

- Health-related news articles and blogs
- Photos and videos that evoke healthy living—your own or repins
- Life-saving self-exam diagrams for skin cancer, breast cancer, and more
- Stress-reducing images and advice
- Sleep articles and blogs
- Diagrams highlighting the benefits of certain exercises (endorphin-boosting, fat-burning, etc.) and the calories each one burns

"The difference between the possible and impossible lies in the person's determination." —Anonymous

5: Favorite Products Board

Finally, create a board to pin everything that appeals to you in terms of gadgets, equipment, must-haves to buy when you reach your goal, and any other material items that strike your fancy. This is the really fun part. It's all about you and customizing to your favorites. Think of it as a virtual shopping spree. You might decide to pin healthy kitchen tools like misters that let you spray flavored oils on your salad to cut calories without losing flavor or crispness. Or you could pin a list of the year's hottest new electronic devices to help you track and measure your fitness level.

Feel free to pin any products that make you look and feel happier and healthier, from makeup to music. It's a great place to find healthy gift ideas, too.

To find ideas, start by checking out Mitzi's Favorite Products Board. For example, I love the Ove Glove, so of course I've got it on my board. It's a five-fingered heat-resistant glove you can use with either hand for putting foods in the oven, getting them out, or manning the grill without getting burned. I've also pinned useful gadgets like an avocado cuber, a Crock-Pot Lunch Crock to take to work, and my favorite multivitamin.

Be Polite: Pinterest Etiquette Pointers

Give credit. If you upload an image you find online, be sure to link to the page where you found it. If you realize that another Pinterest user has neglected to provide a link to a source, send them a polite comment encouraging them to do so.

Be respectful. Leave positive, encouraging comments—not negative, critical ones. If you dislike or disagree with someone's pins, don't follow them.

Stay alert. If you see inappropriate or negative pins, click on the flag icon or the "Report Pin" button to let the Pinterest staff know that a fellow user's conduct is questionable.

Courtesy of Pinterest.com

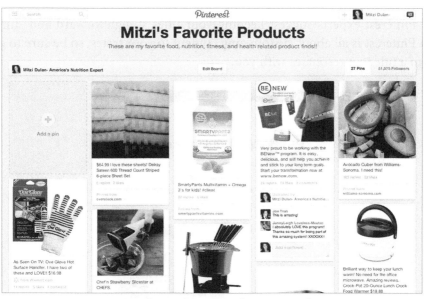

Mitzi's Favorite Products Board

What to pin:

- Kitchen tools and gadgets
- Fitness equipment
- Spa and bath items
- Makeup and beauty products (anti-aging recommendations are always welcome)
- Take-along containers for healthy snacks
- Easy-to-carry water bottles
- Interesting nutrition products
- Flattering, moisture-wicking workout pants
- Tabata timer for your workout
- New smaller plates you want to buy at Crate & Barrel to reduce calorie intake

What's In A Name?

Use the names I've suggested for your five life-transformation boards. It will help you properly follow *The Pinterest Diet*. But feel free to create additional Pinterest boards—as many as you like.

Pinterest experts suggest keeping your titles straightforward and simple. But Pinterest is all about customizing content to your tastes, so be sure to give them a title that resonates with you.

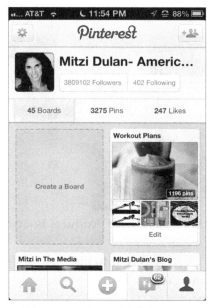

Pinterest On A Mobile App

Remember! Pin 10!

Set aside at least 10 minutes every day to devote to pinning. I've found that time blocking works best for me. Set a timer on your iPhone or smartphone for 10 minutes. Then, pin away! Do this two to three times a day, if you like.

It's easy to pin anywhere if you upload the Pinterest mobile app to your phone, whether you're waiting at the doctor's office or filling time during your kid's soccer practice. With so much new and interesting health and fitness content being created, you'll have a constant supply of great recipes, workouts, articles, and inspiration. One of the things that I love most about Pinterest is that even if I'm browsing the Internet during a non-Pin 10! time, if I find a fantastic article and want to keep it for future reference I just pin it to my In The Know Board. Love this!

Most importantly, spend time on your boards. Admire the beautiful images. Glance through the helpful hints to refresh your memory. Read the motivational quotes to refocus yourself on your goals.

Pin It: Mitzi's Top Twelve

In addition to discovering delectable recipes on many food blogs, I find an unending stream of clean-eating recipes, workout plans, interesting articles, and words of inspiration on the following 12 websites.

1. Shape.com
2. FitSugar.com
3. WomensHealthMag.com
4. Greatist.com
5. Self.com
6. OxygenMag.com
7. CleanEatingMag.com
8. CookingLight.com
9. Health.com
10. MuscleandFitnessHers.com
11. FitnessMagazine.com
12. MensHealth.com

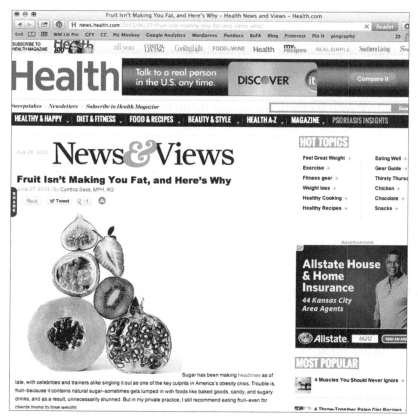

Sample Health.com Article With Pin It Button

How To Unfollow A Pinner

Once in a while, you'll decide to follow a fellow pinner only to find that his or her pins are negative or simply not what you need. Here's how to keep them from popping up the next time you log onto Pinterest:

1. Go to the person's profile by clicking on their name from a pin or board.
2. Click "Unfollow All" to unfollow all of their boards or click "Unfollow" on specific boards of theirs that you want to stop following.

Source: Pinterest.com

Going Solo

Pinterest lets you create up to three "secret" boards that are yours alone as well as public boards that other Pinterest users can see and repin. To make sure a board is for your eyes only:

1. Click your name in the profile menu to go to your profile.
2. Scroll to the bottom of your boards.
3. Click Create a secret board.
4. Choose a name and category for your board. The secret setting will already be set to "Yes."

Any time you add a new board, you can switch the secret setting to "Yes" to make it exclusively yours. Just remember, you can't change a board that you've already created as "public" a secret board.

Source: Pinterest.com

Do It Yourself: Uploading Your Own Content

Here's how to upload a pin from your computer:
1. Take a photo with your digital camera and upload it to your computer, saving it as a JPG, PNG, or GIF.
2. Log onto Pinterest. Hover over the profile menu and click "Upload a pin."
3. Click "Choose File" and find the photo file on your computer.
4. Choose the board you want to pin to and add a description to your pin.
5. Click "Pin it."

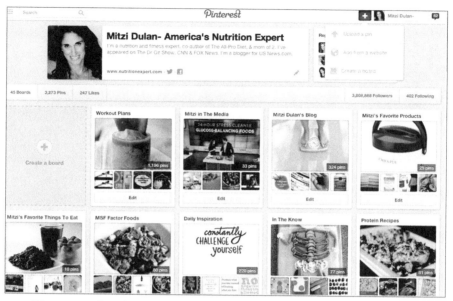

How to Upload A Pin, Add From A Website Or Create A Board

Word to the wise: Pinterest doesn't display high-resolution images. You can upload them, but the full quality won't transfer to the Pinterest site.

More options:

On the go? You can download apps that let you pin photos directly from your iPhone, iPad, Android, or other mobile device.

Want cool effects? There are a number of free websites that allow you to upload photos from your computer, add fun text treatments, then pin them. For instance, PinWords.com lets you upload a photo and type in inspirational quotes with fun effects that look handwritten, taped, or typed on an old-fashioned typewriter. Two more cool websites:

- PicMonkey.com allows you to edit photos, add text, and create collages and then post them to Pinterest.
- Pinstamatic.com lets you create pins from quotes, add text to photos, and more.

CHAPTER 3:

THE PINTEREST DIET RULES

"Don't let the past steal your present."
—Cherralea Morgan

n this chapter, I'll walk you through the 12 essential rules of *The Pinterest Diet*. Don't worry. They're easy to understand and simple to follow. Just remember, you've got to stick to all of them every day to make *The Pinterest Diet* work for you. This is one time when rules are NOT meant to be broken!

Rule #1: Create Your Five Transformation Boards.

In chapter two, you learned everything you need to know about building your 5 Transformation Boards on Pinterest. They're the cornerstones for all the amazing discoveries and triumphs you'll enjoy on your journey to a better body. Once you've created your boards, you'll have everything you need to succeed neatly organized in one convenient, easy-access spot. You can log on wherever and whenever you need support, guidance, or encouragement—during your lunch hour at work, when you're standing in line at the grocery store, if you're debating what to order at a restaurant, or if you're wrestling with a sudden fit of the midnight munchies. Create these five transformation boards now if you haven't already. There's no time like the present to stop wishing for that new body and start working toward it.

Rule #2: Pin 10 Minutes Every Day.

One of Pinterest's best features is its dynamic nature. It's always changing, always expanding and improving. Your Transformation Boards should be all set. You should add to at least one board every day. Better yet, pin new material to all five!

Pinterest is an endlessly rich source of great material, so mine it. Remember! Pin 10! Spend at least 10 minutes EVERY SINGLE DAY combing through Pinterest, looking for great new recipes, exercises, inspirational quotes, health tidbits, products, and anything else that strikes your fancy. Spend a lot of time scouring my boards. At the time I wrote this book, I had more than 3,200 pins to choose from. I've already curated for you, collecting what I consider the best health, fitness, and inspirational material available on Pinterest.

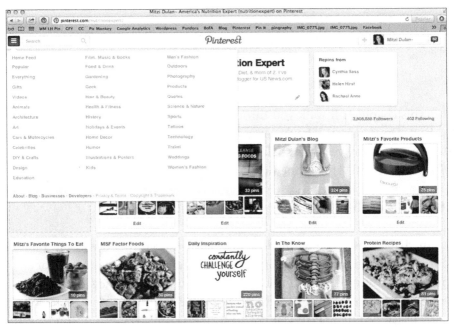

Use Search Categories To Find New Pins

Are the leaves beginning to turn gold and the air suddenly getting crisp and chilly? Search Pinterest for some fresh fall ideas: a list of fun autumn workouts you can do outdoors; beauty tips to protect your skin in cool weather; and healthy treats featuring fruits and veggies that are at their peak of ripeness in September and October, like oatmeal-apple-raisin treats or grilled pears with honey.

Are the November and December holidays approaching, bringing with them a houseful of guests and a seemingly endless stream of parties? Let Pinterest help you plan ahead with a list of tasty, healthful foods you can eat without sabotaging your weight-loss goals, helpful hints of handling holiday stress, or clever ways to get visitors to pitch in with cooking and cleanup. Pinterest can also give you an enormous number of decorating ideas for parties.

Is beach season around the corner? Let Pinterest help you find the most slimming swimsuit styles, great hip- and leg-toning workouts, and the latest news on protecting your skin from the sun's rays.

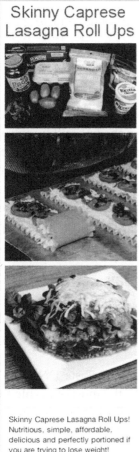

Skinny Caprese Lasagna Roll Ups

Skinny Caprese Lasagna Roll Ups! Nutritious, simple, affordable, delicious and perfectly portioned if you are trying to lose weight! #healthyrecipes #client

3,153 repins 478 likes 9 comments

Uploaded by:
Mitzi Dulan- America's Nutritio...

A Sample Pin

Think about what you've been feeling this week. If you've been craving chocolate, check my boards and do a quick Pinterest search for healthy cocoa bean-based snacks. And don't forget to check the recipe chapter of this book. I've included some mouthwatering ideas for occasional indulgences. If you've been feeling frazzled and overwhelmed, maybe it's time to add a few motivational quotes to remind yourself to slow down and unwind along with a five-minute meditation video.

Remember to check my boards and pins regularly for new nutrition and fitness plans, recipes, quotes, tips, tricks, and more. As you know by now, I'm a Pinterest junkie. I'm always updating my boards with great information I've created myself or pinned from other trustworthy sources.

TIMER TRICK: Set aside a 10-minute block of time and set the stovetop, phone or computer timer to keep track. Log out of email. Don't answer the phone. Don't snack. Forget about your To Do list. Don't let yourself get distracted. Do nothing but pin. Slow down, focus on the task at hand, and let yourself enjoy pinning.

By spending time pinning, you're taking care of yourself. You're nourishing your creativity, you're nourishing your mind, and you're nourishing your body. You're also rekindling your determination to reach your goals, and reenergizing yourself. You're giving your brain and body a well-deserved mini-break from the stresses of daily life. Before you know it, you'll start to look forward to your pinning time. If you're like me, it will soon become one of your favorite times of the day.

Speaking of that, you don't have to pin at the same time every day, though creating a routine can be helpful. Experiment with different times. What fits your schedule best? When are you least likely to get interrupted? When do you need motivation most?

If you want to keep going after 10 minutes and you've got the time to spare, go for it. If you want to log on again later, terrific.

Rule #3: Embrace Your Unique Taste DNA.

In chapter five, you'll find out how to identify your personal Taste DNA. Knowing this is crucial in helping you to break free from the unhealthy control that sugar, salt, and fat can have on your cravings, your waistline, and your life. Imagine being able to eat the foods you truly love and lose weight at the same time! Yes, it's possible.

Once you understand your Taste DNA, I'll show you some simple ways to make the right food choices and map out a delicious meal plan that will help you slim down, feel better, and stay satisfied . . . permanently.

Rule #4: Eat Three MSF Factor Foods Every Day.

Tired of the rollercoaster that hurtles you from starving to binging and leaves you feeling guilty and miserable? Then I've got good news for you: You can finally stop playing the dieter's hunger games!

After you've read chapter five, pinpointed your Unique Taste DNA, and identified a range of yummy meals and snacks that make the most of it, rule #4 is easy. Eat three MSF Factor Foods and Meals from my list in your diet every day. Make sure the ones you choose fit your taste profile, whether you love savory, sweet, crunchy, chewy, or smooth foods.

MSFs are nutrient-rich foods high in protein and/or fiber, and/or healthy fats. They keep you satisfied without loading your body up with junk like trans fats, sugar, and empty calories. Another benefit of MSFs is that they help stabilize your blood sugar so you won't crave the unhealthy stuff like sugar and salt.

Check out chapter four for a full list of MSF Factor Foods.

Rule #5: Know Your Protein Goals.

Protein-rich foods are the most filling foods around. They'll keep you feeling full longer than anything else you put in your body. Plus, studies show that eating more protein helps to stabilize your blood sugar level, which means you'll have more and longer-lasting energy. You'll also avoid that shaky, ravenous sick-hungry feeling.

In chapter six, I'll walk you through the basics of figuring out exactly how much protein you need based on your weight. Once you know your protein goals, I'll help you find easy ways to work them into your daily routine. I'll also give you lots of ideas for tasty protein-rich foods and snacks (don't worry, there are plenty that will appeal to vegetarians) and share my favorite tips for sneaking an extra protein punch into some of your favorite dishes.

Rule #6: Cook At Home At Least Twice A Week.

There are so many benefits to making your own meals!

First, when you cook your food, you can control what you put into your body. Unless you sneak into a restaurant's kitchen, you have no idea how much butter, oil, and salt gets secretly slipped into what's on your plate. Likewise, if you eat packaged meals, you're almost invariably loading up on preservatives and artificial additives. Just take a look at the ingredient list on the back of the box and try to count how many mystery words it includes like hexametaphosphate. When you make it yourself, you eat healthier and you consume fewer calories.

Second, cooking at home is budget-friendly. The typical American spends more than $2,500 eating out every year, according to the United States Department of Labor. The average family shells out $4,000 at restaurants annually, according to a recent ABC News report. Worse yet, we spend $1,000 a year on takeout coffee—more than we spend commuting. It's a high price to pay for convenience, and it's a surefire diet saboteur.

You don't have to be Martha Stewart to make healthy, delicious meals at home. Chapter 10 is filled with simple, delicious, nutritious recipes I've created and vetted myself. And you'll find loads more of them on my Pinterest boards. I'm constantly adding to my recipe repertoire, so I promise you'll never get bored. In fact, you literally never have to eat the same dish twice, though you'll undoubtedly find favorites that you'll want to use again and again.

The Pinterest Diet recipes focus on simplicity and delicious flavor. They're also quick and easy enough for even the most inexperienced cook to tackle. To make home cooking even more convenient, check my Pinterest boards. My In The Know Board includes useful cooking information, time-saving tips, and ways to plan ahead that will make cooking a cinch. You'll also find handy hints for modifying recipes to satisfy your Unique Taste DNA, to include MSFs, to showcase the freshest seasonal ingredients, and to avoid allergy triggers.

Got kids? No worries. My two young daughters have tasted all my recipes, so they're all child-approved!

> *"I'm gonna make the rest of my life, the best of my life."*
> *—Anonymous*

Rule #7: Savor Slowly.

One of the keys to *The Pinterest Diet* is to learn to give your food the attention it deserves. That means I want you to eat consciously. (Hint: That doesn't mean sitting on the couch with a bag of chips while you're watching TV.) You'll learn how to stop "unconscious eating," which leads to overeating. Instead, you'll slow down and savor, paying attention to every bite you put in your mouth.

Most of us scarf down our food, especially when we're stressed. That heaps more stress on us and causes us to gain unwanted pounds. When we slow down and pay attention to the process of eating, it helps awaken all our senses. We enjoy food more, we calm down, we digest more effectively, and we eat less.

Here's my favorite way to get started, adapted from the ancient Buddhist technique of mindful eating. I call it The Raisin Test. I was recently a guest nutrition expert on the *Dr. Oz Show* and I actually conducted this raisin test with Dr. Oz's entire studio audience.

1. Sit in your chair and place a raisin in your hand.
2. Look at the raisin closely. Become conscious of what you see. Notice its shape, color, size, and texture. Is it hard or soft? Smooth or rough?
3. Bring the raisin to your nose and smell it.
4. Tune in to your response to it. Do you want to eat the raisin? Is it hard to resist popping it into your mouth?

5. Put the raisin in your mouth and feel it against your tongue.
6. Bite lightly into the raisin, paying attention to what you taste and feel. Is it squishy, chewy, sweet?
7. Chew three times and then stop.
8. Think about the flavor and texture of the raisin.
9. Finish eating the raisin and sit quietly.
10. Breathe and try to fully sense the experience you just had of eating the raisin.

(Incidentally, if you dislike raisins, you can try the same experiment with half a dried apricot, a green olive, or another bite-sized morsel.)

Apply this same slow-savoring technique to one of your meals every day. It might feel awkward at first, but it will gradually enhance your appreciation and awareness of every bite you take.

The Pistachio Principle

Pistachios in the shell are a great mindful snack because they take longer to eat, which encourages you to slow down and pay more attention to each bite you take. Plus, that huge pile of empty shells makes you more conscious of how much you've eaten.

Research showed that snackers consumed 41 percent fewer calories when they ate pistachios in the shell than when they ate shelled nuts. Equally interesting, when the leftover shells were cleared immediately, snackers ate up to 22 percent more.

Rule #8: Eat Clean.

"Clean eating" is one of the biggest trends in nutrition circles today. In the simplest terms, eating clean means steering clear of highly processed and packaged foods that contain artificial ingredients and focusing instead on whole foods like unrefined whole grains, fresh fruits and veggies, fresh herbs, and antibiotic-free protein sources. It also means avoiding artificial sweeteners. When you eat clean, you get better nutrition, you lose weight, you feel better, and you look better because you reduce your salt intake and therefore avoid bloating.

Lots of experts also believe that avoiding the excess calories and refined sugars typical of a poor diet can help you stave off diseases like cancer and better manage chronic conditions like endometriosis, fibromyalgia, and high cholesterol. Think you can't live without diet soft drinks and nachos? People who try eating clean are often amazed to discover that in a short time their cravings for junk vanish. I've even had clients who were long-time diet soda addicts go cold turkey and discover, to their amazement, that diet soda tasted awful to them after several weeks without it.

In chapter seven, I'll show you how to incorporate MSFs (Most Satisfying Foods) into eating clean. You'll learn simple ways to get the greatest benefits— and enjoyment—out of eating wholesome, nutrient-rich foods that pack a big health-boosting, disease-fighting punch.

Rule #9: Don't Eat After 7:30 p.m.

This rule is non-negotiable. Do NOT eat after 7:30 p.m. Not even a small bowl of popcorn or an apple with peanut butter. I've lost more than 25 pounds and kept it off, and one of the secrets of my success was giving up nighttime snacks. To lose weight, you want your body to burn fat when you sleep. But your body can't do that if it's busy digesting the bag of chips you just devoured while you watched the evening news. Late-night eating can sabotage your diet as effectively as a pint of ice cream.

How do you conquer cravings after 7:30 p.m.?

- Don't keep snacks you can't resist in the house. You can't scarf down a handful of cookies if they're not in the cabinet.
- Do something with your hands. Paint your nails, fold some laundry, log onto Pinterest and start pinning. Keep yourself occupied.
- Change your evening routine. If sitting in front of the television or the computer tends to bring on an insatiable urge to munch, limit the time you spend on those activities. Turn off the TV and take a soothing bubble bath or read a book. Move your laptop to another room farther away from the kitchen. Also, only allow yourself to eat at your dining table. You are not allowed to eat in bed, on the couch, or while you're talking on the phone. You can dramatically

improve your weight loss by becoming more conscious of your eating.

- Drink a cup of herbal tea sweetened with honey.
- Practice deep breathing and do some stretches or a little yoga.
- Try appealing to your other senses. Some studies have found that aromatherapy might be able to curb your appetite. And research has shown that it can reduce stress.
- Light a vanilla-scented candle and play some soft music to soothe yourself.
- Write down what you plan to eat tomorrow morning. I love visualizing myself enjoying breakfast the following day.
- Eat healthful dinners with plenty of protein and fiber to keep you feeling full longer.

Rule #10: Include Planned Indulgences.

Food is one of life's great pleasures. Why miss out on the fun? As I often confess to my clients, I don't eat to live. I live to eat! *The Pinterest Diet* is all about celebrating and savoring fun, delicious food. I'll never force you to live with the dreaded three Ds of discipline, denial, and deprivation.

In fact, guilty pleasures are a must . . . but without the guilt. On *The Pinterest Diet*, it's imperative that you include what I call Planned Indulgences, whether it's a crisp, light fruity white wine or a decadent buttery caramel. Believe me, I get it. I love food too. And like you, I've tried my share of diets that required superhuman willpower. Never again. Instead, I'll teach you how to incorporate indulgences into your diet that let you feel cared for and guilt-free rather than punished and deprived.

Rule #11: Drink "Half Your Weight" In Water.

You've probably heard it before, but it bears repeating: Water is the most important nutrient you can give your body! In fact, the human body is made up of nearly 70% water.

Water helps your digestion. It makes it easier for you to absorb important nutrients. It allows you to maintain a normal body temperature. It keeps your kidneys and bowels in good working condition. It prevents your muscles from feeling fatigued, and it plumps up your skin so it looks less dry and wrinkled.

Drink even more when you're working out to replenish and rehydrate the water you lose when you sweat. Drink before you exercise and regularly during your workout. You also get more easily dehydrated when it's hot, in higher altitudes, and as you age.

The Half Your Weight Water Formula: Here's an easy way to calculate the amount of water you should drink every day: Take your total weight in pounds, and divide by two. That's the number of ounces of water you should be drinking every day. For instance, if you weigh 140 pounds, you should drink 70 ounces of water a day. That's a little less than nine glasses of water.

Other liquids like coffee, alcohol, and especially soft drinks do NOT count as part of your day's water intake.

Water also tends to make you feel more full. Drink water with every meal and snack. Put a bottle in your car on the morning drive to work or tuck a small one in your backpack if you're walking. Eat lots of fruits and vegetables; they've got a high water content, so they'll add to your intake.

I'm going to share an amazing cold water secret with you: Drinking 24 ounces of ice water three times a day burns an extra 100 calories! Here's why: It takes energy for your body to raise the temperature of the water you drink from freezing to body temperature. That makes it a bonus calorie burn for you!

I use a tumbler every day to make sure I drink enough water. Why not add a hint of lemon juice or fresh lemon to your water to jazz it up? I also drink a lot of LaCroix Water, a flavored sparkling water with no artificial sweeteners and no calories.

Avoid buying waters with artificial sweeteners. You'll be drinking a high volume of water, and loading up on chemicals isn't good for your health.

Rule #12: Stick To The Pinterest Diet Workout Plan.

If you've spent years working out without getting the results you want and gotten so bored or discouraged that you gave up, *The Pinterest Diet* Workout Plan will jumpstart your metabolism and get you results fast. In chapter 11, I'll show you how to workout smart and burn calories even when you're not exercising. The workout's calorie-torching exercises are portable and require no fancy equipment, so you can do them at home, at the gym, or even in a hotel room if you're traveling.

All you need is 12 to 30 minutes, three to four times each week.

The Pinterest Diet Rules

Clip this page out of the book and keep it handy—in your purse, on your refrigerator, on your nightstand, or someplace else where you can refer to it easily.

1.   Create Your Five Transformation Boards.
2.   Pin 10 Minutes Every Day.
3.   Embrace Your Unique Taste DNA.
4.   Eat Three MSF Factor Foods Every Day.
5.   Know Your Protein Goals.
6.   Cook At Home At Least Twice A Week.
7.   Savor Slowly.
8.   Eat Clean.
9.   Don't Eat After 7:30 p.m.
10. Include Planned Indulgences.
11. Drink "Half Your Weight" In Water.
12. Stick To *The Pinterest Diet* Workout Plan.

Habit Forming

How long does it take to develop a new habit? 21 days. That's the number most often quoted by experts. That means you have to force yourself to stick to a new behavior every day for three straight weeks before it becomes a comfortable part of your daily routine. In that timeframe, your brain actually forms new neural pathways. Some recent studies say the number varies based on the person—as little as 18 days for some, as long as 66 days for others.

Every habit starts with a three-part process called a habit loop. First, a cue automatically tells your brain to do something. The reward from the behavior (for example, the endorphin rush you get after a workout) helps your brain remember the habit loop and triggers it again in the future. The best part? When a behavior becomes a habit, your brain does it without having to put a lot of conscious thought into it. That means you can devote your mental power to other tasks, notes Charles Duhigg in his book *The Power of Habit*.

When you want to start a habit, don't tell yourself you'll have to do it for the rest of your life. That's overwhelming, intimidating, and discouraging for most of us. Instead, tell yourself you're going to try it for three weeks—or the magic 21 days.

The Pinterest Diet Rules For Kids

One of the biggest challenges parents face today is raising healthy children who understand the basics of good nutrition and are willing to eat a variety of wholesome foods. To help you promote healthy eating in your own home, try these 12 tips.

1. **Start early.** It's much harder to change the habits of an eight-year-old than to incorporate healthy habits when your baby is first beginning to eat solid foods. Introduce him or her to an assortment of flavors during the toddler years and continue to add tastes, textures, and flavors each year. Don't get discouraged if your kids wrinkle their noses the first time. Remember, it can take five to 20 exposures to a new food before a kid begins to like it!

2. **Avoid the "kid food" trap.** This is one of my pet peeves. Parents often assume that children should eat "kid foods" rather than "adult foods." There's no such thing! A barbeque shouldn't mean hot dogs for everyone under 18. Kids can eat grilled chicken breasts, too. Raise your expectations. Require your children to eat the same foods you eat. You'll probably be surprised at how much they enjoy what you once dismissed as "adult" choices. When dining out, never limit your child's choices to the kids' menu.

3. **Take them shopping.** The more involved you can get your kids in the process of selecting foods and cooking them, the better. Let them pick their favorite healthy options at the grocery store and help you prepare them at home. You can also let them grow their own garden. If they grow it, they'll be more likely to eat it.

4. **Control what comes into your kitchen.** If you only buy wheat bread, you won't have to worry about your child eating white bread at home. Your kids will get used to whole wheat and whole-grain products, if that's all you serve. You're the adult. *You* decide what food enters your home.

5. **Ban the clean plate club.** Forcing your kids to eat everything on their plate is a bad plan. It reinforces the idea that they should only feel full once they've gobbled up all the food in sight. It teaches them to ignore their body's internal cues of satiety and hunger, which can set them up for a lifetime of overeating.

6. **Refuse to be a short-order cook.** The entire family should eat the same meal, unless there's a medical reason to serve your child a different dish. Moms, you're busy enough! You should never be forced to prepare three different meals to please three different family members. Instead of making special foods for picky eaters, pair a familiar food with an unfamiliar one for everyone.

7. **Strike a balance.** Being too strict can backfire. In fact, I've had many clients who blame their weight struggles on growing up in a restrictive eating environment. Rather than banning pizza and ice cream forever, strive for a happy medium when it comes to healthy eating. Include fun "forbidden" foods occasionally.

8. **Eat dinner as a family.** Sitting down to meals together is good for your kids' health and their happiness. In fact, research shows that pre-teens and teenagers who eat five or more family meals per week have lower rates of smoking, drinking, and illegal drug use than those whose families eat two or fewer meals a week together. No matter how packed your children's schedules get, make meals together a priority.

9. **No yucks allowed.** Make a rule that kids must say, "No, thank you" after taking a bite of a food they don't like, rather than "Yuck!" or "Gross!" or "Eeew!"

10. **Ban sugary drink snacking.** Sipping sugary drinks between meals (after school, before soccer practice, after dance class, etc.) adds unnecessary calories and makes kids less likely to eat well at mealtime.

11. **Cook more at home.** Your entire family will be better nourished and have more quality time together. Get them all to pitch in with cooking and cleanup. You'll raise more conscientious kids and you'll show them that meals are not just mom's responsibility.

12. **Remember, you're a role model.** Whether you mean to or not, you set an example for your children every day. If you eat a variety of healthy foods, they're likely to follow suit. If you load up on junk or balk at new flavors, chances are they will too. Lead by example. Eat a balance of whole grains, high-quality proteins, and healthy fats. And explain to your kids why it's important to eat specific foods. For example you might say, "Make sure you eat some protein to help your muscles get stronger."

CHAPTER 4:

SATISFACTION AT LAST! THE MSF FACTOR

"Your body is the result of the choices you make. Choose right."
—Anonymous

Satiety: One of the hottest *new* buzzwords in weight loss today, satiety (pronounced sa-TI-eh-TEE) simply means being full or satisfied enough that you don't want any more to eat.

You don't reach your goals by saying "no." You get there by saying "yes." And *The Pinterest Diet* is all about yes.

Yours Truly

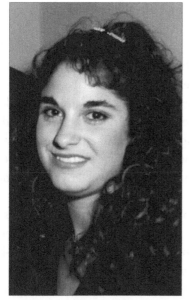

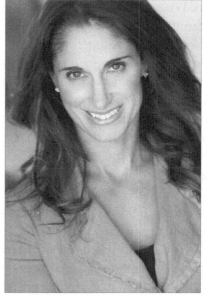

**Before: College Freshman At
148 Pounds**

After: Mom of 2 At 122 Pounds

Yes to food that tastes great.

Yes to food that satisfies your hunger.

Yes to Planned Indulgences.

Satisfying food is the ultimate key to successful weight loss. Which foods make you feel most satisfied? How can you make sure you get plenty of them every day? Answer those questions, and you'll avoid overeating. You'll consume fewer calories, which means you'll lose weight. And you'll do it without feeling hungry or deprived.

I know this approach works because I've used it myself. After years of struggling with my own weight despite all I knew about nutrition and fitness, I got my best body at 33—after having two kids, no less. I've got more energy and I feel healthier and happier with my body than ever! I got there by following the same program I help my clients learn to apply to their daily lives: by focusing on eating satisfying foods.

Your Brain On A Typical Diet

Let's take a look at what happens inside your body when you're hungry. You have a command center in your brain that tells your body when you're hungry and when you've had enough. The hypothalamus, as the command center is called, controls your appetite through two hormones—ghrelin and leptin. When your stomach is empty and growling, ghrelin kicks in, triggering that familiar "I'm hungry" sensation.

Now, here's the interesting part: The reason so many traditional diets fail is because they rely on food deprivation and leave you with an empty stomach that sends your body's ghrelin release into overdrive. Ghrelin—the "I'm hungry" hormone—floods your system, making you want to gobble up everything in sight. The result? You're miserable, frustrated, and famished the whole time you're on the diet. You're pitting your mind against your body and probably chiding yourself for your lack of "willpower." The truth is, no rational, reasonable person has that kind of superhuman willpower anyway. It's not a sensible solution to weight loss.

On the other hand, eating foods rich in fiber, protein, and healthy fats can stimulate the satisfaction hormone, leptin. Leptin is the chemical messenger that tells your body when you've had enough. Think of ghrelin as the green-light hormone and leptin as the red-light one, signaling you to stop eating.

Unfortunately, many highly processed foods aren't rich in these important nutrients. That means your appetite doesn't shut off and neither do your cravings. No wonder it's so tempting to down an entire bag of cookies in one sitting! Countless chronic dieters have spent years beating themselves up over their inability to resist things like doughnuts and cheese puffs. But it's not about willpower! It's about nature. Your body isn't programmed to handle highly processed foods. They can short-circuit your natural appetite shut-off switch. (Not to mention the fact that they're bad for your health and your waistline.)

The Pinterest Diet offers a much more sensible approach to lasting weight loss: Just let your body do what it naturally wants to do. Feed it good, healthful, tasty foods. These are the foods that have what I call a high MSF Factor—Most Satisfying Food Factor. And they're the foods that will help you to feel satisfied. Satiety research has long been an interest of mine, so I'm thrilled to see it getting more attention. In addition to helping satiety individually, when you combine protein, fiber, and fat together they increase satiety through food synergy.

MSF foods help to stabilize your blood glucose levels and help you feel satisfied. Before you know it, you'll find yourself eating less, feeling satisfied, and shedding pounds. Believe it or not, your body will stop sending you messages to wolf down bags of chocolate chip cookies. (Your arteries will thank you for it, too.)

The MSF Factor

Have you ever felt ravenous an hour after your morning bagel and coffee? Ever sink into a low-energy slump that strikes around 3 p.m.? Ever polish off a whole plate of pasta only to end up unsatisfied and craving something more? Who hasn't? And very often, the problem is that the food choices you're making are simply bad at satisfying your hunger.

Protein, fiber, and healthy fats are the best weapons you can give your body to fight hunger. They fill you up, decrease hunger pangs, and keep you feeling full and satisfied longer than carbohydrates alone. They also give you more energy or, as I call it, "staying power." And, because they're not full of refined carbs or sugars, they won't trigger a sugar crash that leaves you feeling sluggish.

The key is to eat at least three MSF Factor Foods EVERY day. MSF Factor Foods contain protein, fiber, healthy fats or a combination of all three. It was tough to narrow the list down to 50, but I picked the superstars—those that pack the biggest nutritional punch and provide the greatest satiety. A few other foods made the list not for their protein, fiber, or fat content, but because they have a high satiety factor. Watermelon, for example, is loaded with water (92% water content), which helps you feel satisfied. And before you panic at the sight of coconut oil on the list, you should know that many experts have changed their mind about it. The newest research shows it's one of the healthiest oils you can eat. Even though 92% of the fatty acids in coconut oil are saturated, they are a healthier class of fatty acids called medium-chain triglycerides (M.C.T.s).

"The difference between your body this week and next week is what you do for the next seven days to achieve your goals."
—Anonymous

Mitzi's Top 50 MSF Factor Foods

Almonds/almond butter
Amaranth
Apples
Avocados
Barley

Bananas
Beans

Blackberries
Blueberries
Cabbage
Carrots
Cheese, natural
Cherries, tart
Chia seeds
Chicken breast, skinless
Coconut oil
Cottage cheese, 1%
Crustaceans
    (crayfish, lobster,
    prawns, shrimp)
Eggs
Extra virgin olive oil
Kamut
Kiwifruit

Lean beef
Lentils
Mackerel
Milk, 1% organic
Mollusks
    (clams, mussels, oysters, scallops)
Oats
Peanuts/peanut butter
and other nut butters
Pears
Pecans
Pistachios
Prunes
Pork tenderloin
Quinoa
Raspberries
Salmon
Sardines
Spinach
Strawberries

Sweet potatoes
Tuna
Quinoa
Walnuts

Greek yogurt	White-fleshed fish
	(cod, flounder, halibut, pollock)
Jerky, natural	Watermelon
Kale	Whole wheat pasta and bread

1. Protein

Call it the keystone for good health. Every cell in your body contains protein. It's in your skin, muscles, internal organs, almost all your bodily fluids—and your body needs regular infusions of it throughout the day to repair damaged cells and to make strong new ones so you can stay healthy.

Protein is one of the best weapons you can give your body to fight hunger. According to a study in the *American Journal of Clinical Nutrition*, protein is more effective at increasing satiety than fat or carbohydrates, it decreases hunger sensations, and it keeps you feeling full and satisfied longer. A recent study from Purdue University also showed that a higher protein diet group enjoyed happier overall moods and more feelings of pleasure than those on other types of diets.

So, if you want to be happier when you're trying to lose weight, aim to make about 30% of your diet protein. Don't worry about the percentage. I'll help you calculate your protein needs in the next chapter and share a detailed list of protein content in popular foods.

Stick to lean protein sources and fatty fish. Some of the best are skinless chicken breast, pork tenderloin, lean beef, salmon, and sardines. Limit your intake of high-fat protein (the kind that comes from a rib-eye steak and whole milk).

Lean protein sources also help your body build and rebuild muscle tissue, provide you with iron to reduce your risk of anemia, strengthen your immune system, and keep your energy level on an even keel. (Remember that when you're shedding pounds, it's especially important to get enough protein to avoid accidentally losing muscle mass.)

Good sources of protein include:
- lean meats, poultry, and fish
- legumes (beans, peas, and lentils)
- eggs
- nuts and seeds
- low-fat milk and cheese products
- whole grains

You'll find out lots more about protein—and the crucial role it plays in healthy weight loss—in the following chapter: Protein Power.

2. Fiber

Soluble fiber—the kind your body can digest—helps lower blood cholesterol and glucose levels. Insoluble fiber—the kind that just passes through your system—improves the health of your digestive system. Equally important if you're watching your waistline, high-fiber foods tend to be lower in calories than low-fiber ones and require more chewing time. You can't wolf them down as easily as you can processed foods, so you're less prone to bingeing when you eat them. Because fiber-filled foods slow digestion, they help you to feel fuller longer and to consume fewer calories throughout the day.

White bread, white rice, white pasta, and anything else made with white refined flour, from cereals to pancake mixes, are generally low in fiber.

> **Did you know?** A 2009 study showed that people who chewed almonds 40 times felt more satisfied and less hungry two hours later than those who chewed their almonds 25 times. So, remember to chew your food slowly and to enjoy every bite.

Here's the ugly truth about what happens when you load up on them: Your body gets flooded with sugar. This is followed by a release of insulin, which causes a sharp decline in your blood-glucose (blood sugar). The insulin moves the sugar from your blood to your liver and muscles, and can also store some as fat. Once the sugar has been processed and your blood-glucose level drops, your energy level plummets, leaving you weak, shaky . . . and famished once more. Repeating the sugar rush–insulin surge cycle several times a day, day after day, week after week, month after month, and year after year sets the stage for insulin resistance and, possibly, type 2 diabetes.

Good sources of fiber include:
- fresh fruits
- fresh vegetables
- whole grains
- legumes (beans, peas, and lentils)

3. Healthy Fats

For years, health and fitness gurus—and even doctors—urged people to avoid fats altogether. But the fat-free philosophy was doomed to fail. Why? Because too often low-fat translates into "tasteless." You end up eating more and feeling less satisfied. Fat was often replaced with more sugar so you didn't save many calories. Stop fearing fats and learn to tell the good ones from the bad. Be aware that there are many different types of fat and that your body will make its own fat if you consume excess calories.

Good fats (monounsaturated and polyunsaturated fats) provide your body with essential fatty acids, which you need for healthy brain function, blood clotting, vitamin absorption, and to prevent inflammation. They're the most concentrated source of calories you can get, which means they give you energy. Including them in your meals helps you feel full and fight the munchies. Good fats can reduce inflammation, too. They're also part of every cell membrane in your body and they play an important role in healing and repair.

Every healthy diet includes them.

Trans fats are the "bad" fats you should avoid. Trans fat raises your "bad" (LDL) cholesterol and lowers your "good" (HDL) cholesterol. What is a trans fat? Trans fats are created by adding hydrogen to vegetable oil through hydrogenation. Fast foods tend to be steeped in trans fats, as are baked goods like doughnuts and Danishes. Food manufacturers have been working to take trans fats out of their products, and, as of 2006, companies were required to list trans fat content on the nutrition facts label. But you should still read labels carefully! In the U.S., if a food has less than 0.5 grams of trans fat per serving, the label doesn't have to include any mention of trans fat. As you read labels, look for words like "partially hydrogenated" vegetable oil. It's another term for trans fat. Your goal should be to have a zero intake of trans fats.

Saturated fats are trickier, because they're not all created equal. In general, you should limit your saturated fat intake since it typically raises total blood cholesterol and "bad" (LDL) levels, increasing your risk of cardiovascular disease and possibly type 2 diabetes. A note about cholesterol in foods: although cholesterol-containing foods have long been blamed for high cholesterol levels, researchers have now found that the biggest influence on your blood cholesterol levels, in addition to heredity, is the amount of trans and saturated fat in the diet.

Healthy fats like **monounsaturated** and **polyunsaturated fats** help to lower both blood cholesterol levels and triglyceride levels. Research has linked monounsaturated fats to reducing belly fat and improving health. **Omega-3** fatty acids are one type of polyunsaturated fat. They include eicosapentaenoic acid (EPA), docosahexaenoic acid (DHA), and alpha-linolenic acid (ALA). Research has shown that including them in your diet can improve your heart health and stave off inflammation. Omega-3s are found in fatty fish, sardines, walnuts, flaxseeds, and chia seeds, though the plant-based sources aren't as effective as fatty fish in reducing heart disease risk. That means you need fish and often fish oil supplements to get enough omega-3s.

Because omega-3s provide so many benefits for heart health, the American Heart Association (AHA) has come out with the following recommendations:

- Healthy adults should consume fatty fish twice a week.
- People with coronary heart disease should consume 1000 mg of EPA plus DHA daily from oily fish. (Talk with your doctor about taking supplements to meet these levels.)
- People with elevated triglycerides, who are under a physician's care, might benefit from taking 2 to 4 grams of EPA plus DHA per day, but should consult a doctor first.

A word of warning: Scientists have found elevated mercury levels in some fish and fish products. The highest are in fish that eat other fish, including shark, swordfish, king, mackerel, and tilefish. If you eat a lot of fish, get your mercury levels tested.

Because skipjack (light) tuna contains one-third the amount of mercury found in albacore (white) tuna, the Environmental Protection Agency states that it's safe to eat up to 12 ounces of light tuna a week. If you can't resist white tuna, eat no more than six ounces a week (the standard weight of one can). Sticking to this limit is especially important for pregnant women. If you're expecting, I'd advise avoiding swordfish, king mackerel, shark, and tilefish altogether.

To learn the mercury levels of various species of fish, check out the Natural Resources Defense Council website at nrdc.org/health/effects/mercury/guide.asp. To find out more about safe levels of tuna, go to the Environmental Working Group's website at ewg.org/tunacalculator.

To play it safe, switch from fish that tends to be high in mercury to fish with lower levels, such as salmon, sole, shrimp, herring, or haddock. I encourage my clients to steer clear of shark and swordfish.

If you're not getting enough omega-3s from food sources, I recommend taking fish oil supplements. Be careful though. Taking three to four grams of fish oil a day can have potential blood-thinning effects, so discuss supplements with your physician.

Fat Guidelines

- Aim to eliminate trans fats from your diet. Avoid fried fast foods and commercially baked goods, and read food labels carefully.
- Eat at least one source of omega-3 fats daily. Sardines, salmon, and walnuts contain omega-3s.
- Include the following sources of healthy fats in your diet:

Monounsaturated fats:

- Almond, avocado, macadamia nut, olive, and sesame oil
- Avocados
- Chocolate
- Nuts and nut butters (almonds, peanuts, macadamia nuts, hazelnuts, pecans, cashews)
- Olives

> **Did you know?** Avocados act as a "nutrient booster." When you eat them with other nutrient-rich foods, they enable your body to absorb more nutrients from the other foods.

Polyunsaturated fats (including omega-3s):

- Chia seeds
- Fatty fish (salmon, tuna, mackerel, herring, trout, sardines)
- Flaxseed, hempseed, sesame, and walnut oil
- Sunflower, sesame, flaxseed, hemp, and pumpkin seeds
- Walnuts

The Power Of Paper And Pen: Your Food Journal

According to the National Weight Control Registry, people lose weight more successfully and maintain their weight loss better when they write down what they eat.. Putting it on paper makes you accountable. It's a lot like keeping track of your checking account balance: jotting down everything that goes in and everything that comes out is the only accurate way to keep track of it.

Here's a simple exercise to get you started: Write down everything you ate today. I have a handy food log you can download on my website at NutritionExpert. com. Use it. Even if you miss a day or a meal here and there and have to leave a few blanks. If you can remember, write down everything you've had for breakfast, lunch, dinner, and snacks for the past two days. You don't have to be too specific; a rough estimate will do. If you can't remember what went in during the past 24-48 hours (or if you'd rather not), start from your next meal.

I ask every one of my clients to do the same. They keep a record of all the food and drink they've had for three to five days before our first visit. If you're like them, you'll probably find that when you review your menu from memory instead of writing it down as you go, you contract caloric amnesia: You forget all about the pretzels you munched on while you scanned the fridge for a snack and the bits of cheese you ate as you prepared that yummy lasagna for dinner. You conveniently block out the fact that the last half of your child's order of fries ended up in your stomach instead of hers (or the garbage or the leftover drawer in the fridge). Don't worry. You're not alone. Most of us tend to grossly underestimate how much we actually eat!

As you look over the meals and snacks you listed, ask yourself how much of your diet generally comes from carbs. How much comes from protein? How many of your meals generally include protein? How many of your snacks do? Your goal should be to include a minimum of 15 grams of protein for breakfast, 30 grams for lunch and dinner.

Remember—no one has to see your food log but you. It's like your diary. Get a lock and key if it helps.

Success Story: Bryan Busby

It was almost four years ago when Bryan Busby, chief meteorologist for KMBC-TV Channel 9 Evening News in Kansas City, and I starting working together to help him shed weight and shape up.

Even though Bryan's career is in the public eye, his primary concern wasn't his appearance, but his health. Bryan had been diagnosed with Type 2 diabetes eight years earlier, and his blood sugars weren't well controlled when we met, even with medication.

My first step was to ask Bryan to start keeping a food journal. I was curious to know not only what he ate and drank—but *when*. He worked from about 2 p.m. until 11 p.m., the same hours as most of the Kansas City Royals players I'd worked with, and I had a hunch that he was grappling with the same problem I'd seen in so many of them.

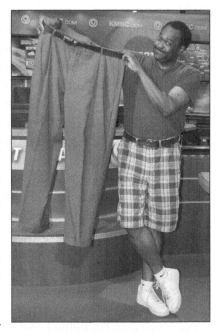

Photo by Mark Lea

Sure enough, Bryan ate very little in the mornings. Meanwhile, his calorie intake in the evening was very high—especially right before he went to sleep. No wonder he was having trouble losing weight and staying healthy!

I gave him an individualized nutritional assessment and explained the importance of curbing late-night eating to fight fat effectively. I also stressed the importance of eating a healthy breakfast to get his metabolism into gear early in the day.

Together we began brainstorming on ways to improve his nutrition, slash his calorie intake, and get him into a regular exercise routine he could enjoy and sustain. Bryan started eating more fruits, vegetables, protein, whole grains, and Greek yogurt. Spinach, kiwifruit, and endive became some of his favorite foods. His cooking skills also improved as he learned to bring out the flavors without piling on salt or fat.

Fast forward six months, and Bryan was 28 pounds thinner. He had gone from wearing 38" pants to a loose-fitting 34". He'd even donated eight bags of clothes from his bigger days to Goodwill. Most important of all, he had gotten his blood sugar under control.

"Working with Mitzi was a life-changing experience for me," Bryan says. "I hadn't weighed less than 200 pounds since 1994. I've got more energy, I feel more vibrant, I focus better, and, when I have to go on-air for several hours in a row due to severe weather, I don't feel like I need to take a break."

"One of the keys to my success is that I haven't been bored with the food I'm eating," he adds. "I really enjoy experimenting with different foods and flavors like Cajun rubs and other delicious herbs and spices."

But the biggest key to Bryan's success has been getting rid of the typical three Ds of dieting (discipline, denial, and deprivation) and giving himself permission to include Planned Indulgences in his life.

"I might stumble for a meal or a day, but I immediately get right back on track. I don't feel guilty, so I'm able to continue my success," he says.

Even today, KMBC viewers often stop Bryan to ask him the secret of his impressive weight loss. He tells them, "Don't deny yourself all the foods that you love and don't view it as a diet. It has to be a lifestyle approach for the greatest success! And don't say you can't do it because if you want to do it bad enough you can. I'm living proof!"

Portion Know-How

Most of us have portion distortion. What we think of as a "helping" of pasta is actually more like TWO . . . or even THREE portions. On *The Pinterest Diet*, you'll need to manage your portions to reach your goals. Fortunately, it's simple and your portions will be generous enough to keep you feeling satisfied.

Here's how to eyeball your portions to know whether you're eating the right amounts.

Food	Single portion size	As big as . . .
Beans (cooked)	½ cup	A computer mouse
Butter	1 teaspoon	A small postage stamp
Cheese	1 ounces	4 dice
Frozen yogurt	½ cup	A computer mouse
Meat, poultry, or fish	3 ounces	A deck of cards/the palm of your hand
Pasta	1 cup	A baseball
Peanut butter	2 tablespoon	A golf ball
Rice	1 cup	A baseball

Fortunately, more food companies and restaurants now offer portion-controlled options to make things easier. (Check my Pinterest boards regularly. I'm always adding more as I find them!) Look for your favorite wholesome foods at the grocery store in portion-controlled packaging with the calories pre-counted.

Here are some more of my top strategies for keeping your portions under control.

1. **Pre-portion your food.** Do this for any foods that come in packages larger than single-serving helpings.
2. **Plan ahead.** Figuring out what you're going to eat in advance helps you control your portions. If you'll be cooking at home, choose the amount to prepare. If you'll be eating out, check the menu online beforehand to identify the smartest choices. If you're going to a party, don't go when you're ravenous. Eat a little protein (a few slices of nitrate-free deli meat with a light cheese, for example) beforehand, so you won't gobble up whatever you see at the party.

3. **Share it**. This strategy comes in handy at restaurants. Split an appetizer or even an entrée with family or friends when you dine out. If you're eating out alone, order a protein-packed appetizer for your meal, like ahi tuna or grilled chicken skewers. If that's not available, ask your waiter to bring you half and put the rest in a to-go bag so you won't be tempted to devour it too.

4. **Use smaller dishes.** Research shows that people eat less when they eat from smaller bowls and plates. Unfortunately, dishware sizes have expanded over the past 20 years almost as much as waistlines have. If you're among the 54 percent of Americans who clean their plates, consider replacing your plates and bowls with smaller ones—or use salad plates as dinner plates.

5. **Ban serving bowls from the table.** Control your environment by making it harder to grab second helpings. Portion out your meal and immediately put the leftovers in food storage containers, so you won't be tempted to overeat.

6. **Add healthy ingredients to your recipes.** Including vegetables in the dishes you cook at home pumps up their nutritional value—and gives you more to eat—without adding a lot of calories. Fresh herbs and spices also tend to make your food more flavorful and satisfying without adding calories.

7. **Establish approved eating areas in your home.** Think about where you consume most of your calories at home. On your couch? In bed? Allow yourself to eat ONLY when you're sitting down at your table or on a stool at your kitchen counter. It might be a challenge at first, but it's the best way to put a permanent stop to unconscious overeating.

8. **Eat consciously.** Make it a habit to eat sitting down, chewing slowly, and savoring your food. Make the most of the portions you've given yourself. If you're having trouble, try the raisin test again. (It's in chapter three, if you need a refresher!)

Your Calorie Budget

In some ways, weight loss is like a math game. Calorie counting gets a bad rap, but it's essential. If you want to lose weight, you have to burn off more calories than you take in. If you want to maintain your weight, you've got to have roughly the same amount of calories coming in and going out.

I call it managing your calorie budget. It's just like managing your financial budget. You have to keep track of how much you take in and how much you expend if you're going to have any control over your weight.

Most of us underestimate the number of calories we eat, just like we underestimate our portion sizes. What you think was a 1600-calorie meal might actually have been closer to 2500 when you add the sauce, the butter, or the gravy.

A sample calorie budget might look like this:

DAILY CALORIE BUDGET

Normal daily calorie intake = 1700
Daily calorie intake needed to lose weight = 1350
Daily calorie budget based on weight-loss goal
Breakfast = 350
Lunch = 450
Afternoon snack = 100 calories
Dinner = 450
If this person had a normal daily intake of 1700 calories and wanted to lose 5 pounds, she could achieve her weight loss by reducing her food intake by 500 calories a day.
1 lb. of fat = 3500 calories
3500 calories/7 days per week = 500 calorie per day reduction of calories. The calorie reduction can come from reducing food intake, increasing exercise, or both. I recommend both. This person could lose 5 pounds in 5 weeks if all she did was reduce her food intake.

One good way to start calorie budgeting is to figure out how many calories you're currently eating on an average day. A great way to see how many calories you're consuming each day is to use MyFitnessPal.com to record your food intake. The site also offers an app that's handy to use and keeps track of your calories as well as your food intake. It's a great tool to help you ensure that you're meeting the protein goals you calculated in chapter six. Or you can start by writing down everything you eat for three days, along with the calorie count of each by looking it up at CalorieCount.about.com. Be ruthlessly honest with yourself. (Remember, you don't have to show the number to anyone else!)

You don't have to be a "perfect" eater to manage your weight successfully. Getting a handle on your calorie budget will help you to get control of your diet—and to budget for occasional indulgences.

Writing down what you eat is not only good for keeping track of calories. It's also a good way to spot trends in your eating habits. Are you gobbling up too many calories from "picking" throughout the day or eating the leftovers from your kids' lunches? Is your diet lacking in fiber or fruit?

Simple Tricks To Help You Budget Your Calories

Lots of the same tactics you can use successfully to control your portions work for calorie-budgeting too. Here are a few more.

- Learn the calorie counts in your favorite foods.
- Read food labels and make smart choices.
- Eat high-fiber foods. They give you more bang for your calorie buck because they keep you satisfied longer and cost you fewer calories.
- Measure out 100-calorie portions of fruits, vegetables, and snacks ahead of time, so you'll have the right amount on hand when you need it.
- Plan your menu for the week. Budget your calories for each day, so you'll be less likely to break the calorie bank.

100 Calories In/100 Calories Out

If you reduce your calorie intake by 100 calories a day or burn an additional 100 calories a day, you'll lose over 10 pounds in a year! Small, steady changes can create big results.

100-Calorie (or Less) Foods

Banana (small) = 100 calories	Chicken breast (2 1/2 oz. grilled) = 100 calories
Greek yogurt (4 oz.) = 100 calorie	Avocado (1/4) = 62.5 calories
Mini Babybel Light (1 disk) = 50 calories	Pineapple (1 cup fresh) = 75 calories
Pretzel crisps: 10 Crisps = 100 calories	Simply Snackin Jerky Treats: 1 serving = 60 calories
Strawberries (1 cup) = 50 calories	Watermelon (2 cups diced) = 100 calories

100-Calorie Burners

(Values are approximate and based on 150-pound person.)	
Beach volleyball: 13 minutes	Cleaning, moderate effort: 26 minutes
Dancing around the living room: 20 minutes	Jumping rope: 9 minutes at a moderate intensity
Mowing the lawn: 20 minutes	Playing with children: 23 minutes
Tennis (singles): 15 minutes	Walking stairs: 11 minutes
Weeding the garden: 18 minutes	Zumba: 11 minutes

5 Ways To Curb Overindulging

Sometimes the urge to binge can hit even when you're not hungry. It might happen because the person sitting next to you at the movies has a tub of buttered popcorn that smells and sounds irresistibly good. Maybe you saw an ad on TV for deep-dish pepperoni pizza and haven't been able to get the mouthwatering image out of your head all day. Here are a few tricks to distract your brain when the desire to overindulge strikes.

1. Stay busy. Focus your attention to something else. Run an errand or head outside to do a quick workout. A change of scenery might be just what you need to distract yourself.
2. Drink water. Hunger can easily be confused with thirst. A tall, refreshing glass of water with a slice of lemon, lime, or cucumber will make you feel less tempted to eat.
3. Have a smart snack. If your cravings strike at a specific time of day, be prepared for them. Pack a tasty calorie-controlled option and eat it a half hour before the old yearning for a visit to the vending machine or the donut shop next to your office kicks in. Try a 100-calorie pack of pistachios (about 30) or two slices of ham with a Laughing Cow Light cheese wedge.
4. Refocus on your goals. Time to turn to your Life Transformation Boards! When the urge to overindulge hits, log onto Pinterest. Check out those great jeans you want to buy (in a size 6!), those toned abs you hope to have by summer, and anything else you're working toward. Will satisfying your craving bring you closer to your goal of losing weight, maintaining your weight, lowering your body fat, toning up, or living a healthier life?
5. Indulge wisely. If you can't resist it any longer, give in . . . but eat a reasonable portion of the food you crave. (Figure out the calorie count ahead of time and eat half. Throw the other half away if you have to.) Eat each bite slowly, taking time to savor it. Afterward, don't waste time feeling guilty. You're human. We all overindulge now and then. Accept it and move on. In fact, indulging your cravings now and then is healthy. Remember, deprivation doesn't work as a diet strategy.

You Drank What?!

Drinking calories is one of the biggest challenges in the American diet today. People are gulping down their calories instead of eating nutrient-rich foods. Unfortunately, most drinks are unsatisfying because they contain very little protein, fiber, or vitamins—or none at all. Equally bad is the fact that most drinks are full of sugar. When I worked with the Golden State Warriors NBA team, I was asked to meet with an injured player so he wouldn't gain weight. I discovered that he drank more than 584,000 calories a year of grape juice! I advised him to stop drinking the juice. To his amazement, he got leaner than he had been in his entire NBA career.

Calories in beverages can add up quickly and sabotage your weight-loss efforts. Here's an eye-opening look at the calorie content in some popular drinks.

100% Fruit Juices:

Apple (8 oz.)	117
Carrot (8 oz.)	98
Cherry (8 oz.)	130
Cranberry (8 oz.)	137
Grapefruit (8 oz.)	101
Orange (8 oz.)	112

Sodas:

Cola (12 oz.)	143
Ginger Ale (12 oz.)	124
Lemon-Lime (12 oz.)	147
Mountain Dew (12 oz.)	165
Orange Soda (12 oz.)	165
Root Beer (12 oz.)	150

Hot Beverages:

Starbucks Caffè Americano (16 oz.)	15
Starbucks Iced Caffè Latte with 2% milk (16 oz.)	180
Starbucks Vanilla Latte with 2% milk (16 oz.)	250

Starbucks Vanilla Bean Crème Frappuccino (16 oz.)	400
(with whole milk and whipped cream)	
Starbucks White Chocolate Mocha with 2% milk (16 oz.)	400
Starbucks Shaken Iced Green Tea (16 oz.)	0

Miscellaneous Drinks:

Fruit Punch (8 oz.)	114
Almond Milk, Sweetened (8 oz.)	70
Fruit Punch (8 oz.)	120
Hemp Milk, Vanilla (8 oz.)	130
Lemonade (8 oz.)	96
Organic 1% Milk (8 oz.)	100
Organic Whole Milk (8 oz.)	150
Red Bull Energy Drink (8 oz.)	108

Specialty Waters:

Coconut Water (20 oz.)	110
LaCroix Sparkling Water (12 oz.)	0
LifeWater (20 oz.)	100
Vitamin Water (20 oz.)	120

Sports Drinks:

Gatorade (20 oz.)	125
Powerade (20 oz.)	75

Alcohol:

Beer (12 oz.)	150
Gin, rum, vodka, whiskey (1½ oz., 80 proof)	100
Gin, rum, vodka, whiskey (1½ oz., 100 proof)	124
Light Beer (12 oz.)	100
Margarita (8 oz.)	540
Rum and Coke (4½ oz.)	150
Wine, red or white (4 oz.)	102

The Pinterest Diet Drinking Rules

During the Jumpstart Cleanse in chapter eight, NO ALCOHOL is allowed. Alcohol can sabotage your weight-loss efforts because it's high in calories and low in nutrition. Plus, when you drink it, your liver has to help process it instead of burning fat, which can lead to more fat storage.

It's common to have a good week of working hard to stick to your diet Monday-Thursday and then, boom! The weekend comes, and you drink too much. And drinking frequently leads to unhealthy eating, because your inhibitions dwindle, your judgment gets impaired, and suddenly eating five pieces of pizza at midnight sounds like a delicious idea.

Keep in mind, if you drink a margarita, you'll be consuming more than 500 calories. It will take you nearly 1½ hours straight of running to burn it off.

Try these tips to limit your consumption:

- Always order a glass of water with your alcoholic beverage. It helps you stay hydrated and provides a feeling of fullness, so you'll drink less.
- Choose drinks with a lower number of calories, but without artificial sweeteners. (In other words, don't order rum and Diet Coke!) Check out my 3 delicious low-calorie alcoholic beverages: Skinny Strawberry Sangria, Skinny Cape Cod, and Skinny Prosecco in the recipe chapter. You can add flavored sparkling water to lower the calorie content of many drinks without adding artificial sweeteners.
- After your 7-Day Jumpstart Cleanse, which you will read about in chapter 8, you can drink in moderation. That means having about one glass a day for women or two glasses a day for men. And balance your calorie budget: Cut back on something else during the day if you plan to enjoy a glass of wine with dinner.

> Did you know? People pour **76%** more into glasses that are short and wide than they do into glasses that are tall and skinny. According to Brian Wansink, Ph.D., short, wide glasses give us a visual illusion of being smaller, so we think we need to fill them up more! Take home message? Choose your glasses carefully. They can wreak havoc on your calorie count if you don't!

CHAPTER 5:

DISCOVERING YOUR UNIQUE TASTE DNA

"The 3 C's of life: Choices, Chances, Changes. You must make a
Choice to take a Chance or your life will never Change."
—Anonymous

Sugar. Salt. Fat. There's nothing "wrong" with modest quantities of these ingredients. All of them are "natural" in their own way. But most Americans' diets include extraordinary amounts of all three. If you eat a lot of highly processed foods, you're probably one of those Americans. And, if so, you've unconsciously allowed your tastes to be reshaped by those foods. When you get used to heaping helpings of sugar, salt, and fat, it's easy to forget what really tastes good to you. In fact, if you eat on the go—wolfing down breakfast on the way to work or hitting fast food drive-throughs—you can reach the point where you hardly taste your food anymore.

But all of us have our own innate personal food preferences. In other words, our own Unique Taste DNA. Certain tastes, textures, and even colors can literally buoy your spirits and make your brain thrum with the thought, "Mmmm, this is good!" You might have that response to a crisp green Granny Smith apple or the salty bite of a well-cured artisanal cheese.

To recognize your Taste DNA, you have to be open to experiencing the vast array of flavors and consistencies that unprocessed foods offer. Some are subtle. Others are strong. Some are complex, some simple.

Finding your Taste DNA can be a source of joy. Once you've discovered it, you start truly tasting your food again. You feel more satisfied after you eat—not inexplicably drawn to the cupboard to rummage for "the right taste." You're also much less prone to emotional eating—munching to stave off the blues or quell your anxieties. Your daily diet choices become much less confusing. In other words, when you know what you like, that's what you eat.

The best way to identify your Taste DNA is to keep a food journal for a week. Don't vary your choices, but slow down and pay attention to the process of eating. Don't watch TV during meals. Don't wash down each bite with a giant gulp of iced tea.

Write down everything you eat. Note where, when, and why you ate it. Were you genuinely hungry or eating for other reasons? Then write down how you felt afterward. Happy? Sluggish? Guilty? Stuffed? Unsatisfied?

At the end of the week, circle the meals and dishes you liked best.

As an alternative to food journaling, just fill out the food chart below.

"Health is the greatest gift, contentment the greatest wealth,
faithfulness the best relationship."
—Buddha.

FOOD FOR THOUGHT: FINDING YOUR FAVORITES

List 5 of your favorite snacks:
1.
2.
3.
4.
5.
List 5 of your favorite appetizers:
1.
2.
3.
4.
5.
List 5 of your favorite dishes for breakfast, brunch, lunch, or dinner:
1.
2.
3.
4.
5.

List 5 of your favorite desserts:
1.
2.
3.
4.
5.
List 5 of your all-time most memorable meals:
1.
2.
3.
4.
5.

Now look at your list or your food journal and see if you notice any trends. To help you pinpoint them, try the following easy exercises.

Step One: Circle all the adjectives below that apply to your favorites.

Acidic	Crumbly	Hot	Smooth
Aged	Crunchy	Juicy	Soft
Aromatic	Dense	Lemony	Sour
Bite-sized	Dry	Light	Spongy
Bitter	Doughy	Mild	Sticky
Bland	Fiery	Moist	Sweet
Briny	Flaky	Nutty	Succulent
Buttery	Fluffy	Peppery	Sugary
Charred	Fresh	Piquant	Syrupy
Cheesy	Frosty	Pungent	Tangy
Chewy	Fruity	Rich	Tender
Chilled	Gamy	Salty	Velvety
Chunky	Garlicky	Silky	Vinegary
Cold	Gingery	Savory	Zesty
Creamy	Gooey	Sharp	Others ____
Crisp	Hearty	Smokey	

Step Two: Circle all the cooking methods that apply to your favorite foods or dishes.

Baked	Grilled	Pickled	Sizzling
Blackened	Glazed	Poached	Steamed
Boiled	Layered	Puréed	Stuffed
Bubbly	Marinated	Roasted	Toasted
Char-broiled	Mashed	Sautéed	Whipped
Others:			

"If you eat what you've always eaten,
you will weigh what you've always weighed."
—Anonymous

Step Three: Circle all the spices and flavorings that apply to your favorite foods or dishes.

(Don't worry if you don't recognize all the names. You don't have to be a foodie to know what tastes you like! You can also add in personal favorite flavorings like Tabasco.)

Adobo	Cinnamon	Lavender	Pistachio
Allspice	Clove	Lemon	Poppy seed
Almond	Cocoa/chocolate	Licorice	Pumpkin pie spice
Ancho chile	Coconut	Lime	Red pepper
Anise	Coriander	Maple	Rum
Apple	Cumin	Marjoram	Saffron
Banana	Dill	Mint	Sage
Basil	Fennel	Mustard	Salt
Black pepper	Garlic	Nutmeg	Sesame
Butterscotch	Ginger	Onion	Tarragon
Caraway	Hazelnut	Orange	Thyme
Cardamom	Honey	Paprika	Turmeric
Cayenne	Horseradish	Parsley	Vanilla
Chicory	Jalapeno	Peanut	Walnut
Cilantro	Jasmine	Peppercorn	Wasabi
Others:			

Step Four: Review. Spend some time looking back over the words you've chosen. Highlight your all-time favorites. They should give you a good idea of your unique Taste DNA. You might realize the desserts that truly satisfy you are all warm, gooey, and chocolaty, for example. Maybe your favorite snacks are all dense, chewy, and salty. Once you know, you can start to look for healthy recipes to pin (as always, start with my Pinterest boards) that will appeal to your Unique Taste DNA. Then, search Pinterest using both your favorite ingredients and recipes as keywords. Collect some for entrees, salads, vegetables, fruits, soups, snacks and desserts, and others for special occasions.

It's also fun to make a separate list of the textures and flavors you dislike. Once you've homed in on those, you can get a better understanding of how to modify recipes which recipes, restaurant choices, and grocery items to avoid—even if they've been prescribed on every other diet you've tried!

Tasty Tips: Beyond Unique Taste DNA

Here are a few more pointers to make your meals even more satisfying:

Color it up. Including a variety of bright, appetizing colors in your meals makes you feel more satisfied. Eating a salad? Toss in some golden roasted almonds or walnuts, sliced avocado, and fresh sliced strawberries or dried cranberries. Likewise a simple salsa of black beans, yellow corn, and fresh tomatoes with vinaigrette can make a tilapia filet more mouthwatering.

Look at your list of favorite meals. Are there certain colors that appeal more to you than others? Does food look more appetizing to you when it's artistically arranged on the plate or when it looks like simple old-fashioned home cooking like Mom used to make instead of art on a plate? (Remember, there's no wrong answer. You're just trying to figure out what appeals most to you!)

Top the table. Setting a tempting table adds to almost everyone's enjoyment of a meal. (And, remember, you should eat your meals at a table—not on a TV tray or your desk or your couch or your bed.) Clear away anything that might distract you from truly savoring your food, whether it's a stack of mail or a laptop.

Again, review your journal. If you haven't already, make a few notes about the setting of the meals you've enjoyed most. What do you remember about the tablecloth, placemats, dishes, table decorations, and the room where you ate? Does candlelight make dinner more enjoyable for you? Maybe it's time to spring for some inexpensive candles. (Choose unscented ones so the aromas don't interfere with the taste of the food.) Does breakfast taste better with sunshine flooding in? If so, could you move your table to a more light-filled spot in the kitchen or dining room? And, of course, there's no better way to improve the ambiance than with good company.

CHAPTER 6:

PROTEIN POWER

"I may not be the strongest I may not be the fastest but I'll be damned if I'm not trying my hardest."
—Anonymous

When people come to me wanting to lose weight, one of the first things we do is to sit down together and look closely at what they've been eating. Usually, they aren't getting the right combination of foods. Often their meal timing is off, too. They eat too late at night or wait too long between meals.

Most common of all, they're overdoing the carbs and not eating enough protein at one or two meals. The result? They feel both famished and frustrated. It's incredible how quickly adjusting their protein intake quells their hunger pangs, gives them the physical and mental stamina they've been lacking, and helps them shed extra pounds without feeling like they're on a diet!

I actually discovered the importance of protein through personal experience. When I was in high school I became a vegetarian. Living in Kansas didn't make it easy. It's a great state, but it wasn't exactly the vegetarian capital of the world (It still isn't!)

I wasn't the kind of vegetarian who loads up on legumes and knows recipes for quinoa. Nobody had even heard of quinoa back then! I was a *bad* vegetarian. The carb-crazed kind. My first job at KFC didn't help. (I know what you're thinking—unlikely start for a weight loss expert, right? But I was only 15, and that was the only place that would hire me.) My job made loading up on mashed potatoes and biscuits all too easy.

By the time I hit my sophomore year of college, I had high triglycerides and, as a result, I weighed 138 pounds (a lot for my frame). Then, when I was 22, an interesting thing happened: I won an internship as the first-ever sports nutrition intern at the Olympic Training Center in Colorado Springs. I was asked to compile nutrition information to be placed on all the tables in the Olympic Training Center Cafeteria explaining why lean red meat is important for athletes. As I set to work on the project, I began to realize I'd been shortchanging my body. The more I learned, the more convinced I was that I needed to bring lean red meat and other protein sources back into my diet. But, wouldn't it be a shame to blow my record after having been so good all these years? Of course, I wasn't being "good" at all. I just thought I was.

After much deliberation, I decided to have one of the lean steaks in the cafeteria, where we ate all of our meals. As they say, the rest is history.

Amazingly, I lost six pounds in the next four weeks and I stopped feeling constantly hungry. The protein left me much more satisfied than my beloved carbs ever had. I also realized that I was no longer preoccupied with food. (I'd thought about what I'd eaten, what I shouldn't eat, and what I would eat next almost constantly when I was shoveling in all those carbohydrates.)

My body fat started shifting as well. I got much leaner. I was working out all summer in the same facility as the athletes (yes, this internship was a total blast) and finally, the work I was putting in with weights, mountain biking, and running began to pay off.

TIP FOR VEGETARIANS: You can certainly meet your protein needs as a vegetarian, but it takes work. Check my Pinterest boards for great meat-free, protein-rich recipes and suggestions for tasty protein sources that don't include animal products.

Years later, I saw my clients fall into the same carb trap, whether or not they were vegetarians. Cindy was a perfect example. She arrived in my office discouraged by countless futile attempts to diet. At 5'5", 155 pounds, she had tried everything, she said, to lose weight. Nothing had worked. I asked her to write down what she ate on a normal day.

I noticed immediately that she wasn't eating any protein at breakfast—just coffee and a bagel every morning. She usually had a salad for lunch, snacked on the typical office carbs (chips, cookies, and candy) during the afternoon, and ate only a small amount of protein at dinner. She felt hungry all the time and often exhausted, especially in the afternoon, not to mention depressed that she couldn't get the weight off. We upped her protein intake to a total of about 115 grams of protein per day from her old total of about 40 grams per day.

I ran into her two days later in the locker room and she was bursting with enthusiasm. For the first time she could remember, she was feeling energetic all day long. Her snack cravings and hunger pangs had vanished, too. "I feel fantastic!" she told me.

By the way, Cindy reached her goal weight easily in a short time, and said she never felt like she was dieting.

Another memorable example of protein power came when I was helping a group of runners prep for their first marathon with The Leukemia Society Team in Training. I was shocked at how many of them were eating very little protein at breakfast, then eating only pasta with red sauce after their training. I explained the importance of eating protein for recovery from endurance sports like running, to maintain lean muscle mass, and to decrease hunger sensations. They followed my advice and their energy levels skyrocketed.

You don't have to be an endurance athlete to reap the same benefits.

Protein can work as well and as quickly for anyone as it did for Cindy and the Team in Training. I've helped countless clients, from pro athletes to ordinary folks, hoping to shape up and shed some pounds, and adjust their protein levels. Increase your protein intake and you'll end up consuming fewer total calories without even realizing it!

Carb Curbing

My rule of thumb for myself and my clients is **never eat a carb-only meal**. You won't believe how much more energy you'll have. And you'll wonder what ever happened to that old, familiar feeling—the sugar crash that left you sluggish after all those carb-concentrated snacks and meals. (Not that you'll miss it!)

Here's what happens when you eat sugars and refined carbs like sodas and muffins made with white flour. Your body realizes immediately that there's been an influx of sugar. It responds to protect itself by releasing the hormone insulin to bring your blood-glucose (blood sugar) level back down to normal. The insulin moves the sugar from your blood to your liver and your muscle cells.Unfortunately, the higher insulin levels can also increase the amount of glucose that gets stored as body fat. Ugh. Who wants to increase their body fat? Most of us are trying to do the opposite!

Once the sugar's been processed and your blood-glucose level drops, your energy level plummets. You may feel weak, shaky, slightly sick, and hungry again. It becomes a vicious cycle of poor energy, hunger, and increased body fat. Sound familiar?

Need more incentive to scrap that carbs-only meal plan you've been on? Your pancreas, the organ that produces insulin, gets overstimulated and overworked every time you load up on refined carbs and sugars without balancing them with protein and fat, both of which slow digestion. Your blood sugar levels rocket up time and time again, and your pancreas has to rush to the rescue like an EMT worker. Over time, there's a good chance you'll develop insulin resistance, which sets the stage for type-2 diabetes and other serious health issues.

"If it doesn't challenge you, it doesn't change you."
—Fred Devito

Good And Bad Protein

In the past decade we've heard enough about high-protein, low-carb or no-carb diets to last us a lifetime. I'm not giving you permission to go out and wolf down a pound of bacon for breakfast, topped off by a double cheeseburger (minus the bun) for lunch and a sirloin steak for dinner. The high-protein/ low-carb diet craze has made people more aware of different protein sources, which is a good thing. But unfortunately some people use the caveman diet approach as an excuse to gobble up protein sources that were full of grease, unhealthy fats, and sodium.

Another problem: Not all carb-shunning diets told people how much to eat, which left the door open for those who wanted to binge on hunks of cheddar all day. Nor did they always emphasize the importance of getting a healthy level of exercise on a regular basis.

Many high protein dieters lose a significant amount of weight at the beginning, but then find it difficult to maintain the lifestyle. (After all, how many bunless burgers can you eat before visions of risotto start dancing through your head?) They get moody and, more often than not, they gain the weight back eventually.

As you've undoubtedly guessed, I'm against very low-carb—and especially no-carb—dieting. My clients typically get about 30% protein, 30% fats, and 40% carbs, with the majority of carbs coming from fruits, vegetables, beans, legumes, and whole grains instead of sugar-laden carbs from packaged and processed foods. Most of the fats are coming from the healthy types.

So, how do you figure out how much protein your body needs? That depends on whether you want to lose weight or maintain your current weight.

Here's a super-simple formula I use whenever I start working with a new client to pinpoint the level of protein they should eat on a daily basis.

To maintain your current weight: 0.65-0.7 gm/lb

To decrease your body fat and/or lose weight: 0.7-0.9 gm/lb

Example:

A 145-pound woman who wanted to lose weight should eat between 0.7 and 0.9 grams of protein per pound of her current body weight.

0.7 x 140 pounds = 98 grams of protein per day

0.9 x 140 pounds = 126 grams of protein per day

That means she should eat approximately 98 to 126 grams of protein each day.

Protein Plan

When you eat . . .	Make your goal . . .
Breakfast	15 grams of protein
Lunch	35-40 grams of protein
Afternoon Snack	10 grams of protein
Dinner	35-40 grams of protein

Protein Chart

Here's an important list showing the protein content of popular, well-known foods.

MEATS/FISH		
SOURCE	PORTION	PROTEIN (in grams)
BEEF		
Beef, top round, broiled	3 oz.	26
Ground beef, lean, cooked	3 oz.	21
PORK		
Ham, lean, roasted	3 oz.	18
Pork loin chop	3 oz.	28
Pork tenderloin	3.5 oz.	28

POULTRY		
Chicken breast, no skin	4 oz.	30
Chicken leg, with skin	1 leg	30
Chicken thigh, no skin	1 thigh	14
Turkey, no skin	3 oz.	25
SEAFOOD		
Halibut, broiled	3 oz.	23
Sardines, packed in water	3 oz.	23
Salmon, broiled	3 oz.	23
Shrimp, large	15	18
Snapper, broiled	3 oz.	23
Tuna in water	3 oz.	25

EGGS		
SOURCE	PORTION	PROTEIN (in grams)
Egg	1 large	6
Egg whites	2	7
DAIRY/NON-DAIRY SUBSTITUTES		
SOURCE	PORTION	PROTEIN (in grams)
Almond milk, vanilla	1 cup	1
Cheese, American	1 slice	6
Cheese, cottage 1%	½ cup	14
Cheese, cream	2 tbsp/1 oz.	2
Cheese, hard	1 oz./1" cube	7
Cheese, Ricotta, part skim	½ cup	14
Hemp milk	1 cup	2
Ice cream	½ cup	5
Ice cream, low-fat	½ cup	4
Milk, nonfat	1 cup	8-10
Milk, 1%	1 cup	8
Rice milk	1 cup	1
Yogurt, Greek	5 oz.	13
Yogurt, frozen, nonfat	½ cup	4
Yogurt, low-fat, plain	1 cup	12

SOY PRODUCTS

SOURCE	PORTION	PROTEIN (in grams)
Soybeans, cooked	1 cup	29
Soy milk, light	1 cup	7
Soy yogurt	1 cup	6
Tempeh	½ cup	16
Tofu, firm	½ cup	20

BEANS AND LEGUMES

SOURCE	PORTION	PROTEIN (in grams)
Beans, baked	1 cup	14
Beans, black	1 cup	15
Beans, garbanzo	1 cup	14
Beans, kidney	1 cup	15
Beans, pinto	1 cup	14
Beans, refried	1 cup	16
Beans, refried, non-fat	1 cup	14
Black-eyed peas	1 cup	10
Hummus	½ cup	6
Lentils	1 cup	18

NUTS/SEEDS

SOURCE	PORTION	PROTEIN (in grams)
Almonds	1 oz.	6
Cashews	1oz.	4
Chia seeds	3 tbsp	5
Hemp seeds	3 tbsp	10
Peanut butter, natural	2 tbsp	9
Peanuts	1 oz.	6
Sunflower seeds	1 oz.	6
Walnuts	1 oz.	7

GRAINS (cooked)

SOURCE	PORTION	PROTEIN (in grams)
Amaranth	½ cup	5
Barley	½ cup	2
Buckwheat	½ cup	3
Bulgur wheat	½ cup	3

GRAINS (cooked)		
Freekeh	½ cup	6
Kamut	½ cup	11
Millet	½ cup	4
Oats	½ cup	3
Quinoa	½ cup	4
Rice, brown	½ cup	3
Rye	½ cup	12

MISCELLANEOUS		
SOURCE	PORTION	PROTEIN (in grams)
Bread, whole wheat	1 slice	2-3
Fruit	1	0-1
Pasta (cooked), whole wheat	1 cup	8
Protein powders (applies to most)	1 scoop	18-22
Tortilla, flour	1- 9"	3
Vegetables, cooked	½ cup	1-2
Yeast, Brewer's	1 oz.	11

Here are three handy rules of thumb.

1. One ounce of turkey, chicken, fish, lean red meat, or pork equals about 7 grams of protein. That means a 5-oz. chicken breast contains about 35 grams of protein.

2. When you're eyeballing portions, remember that three ounces is about the size of a deck of cards or the average size of a woman's palm.

3. When you're reading packaged food labels, check both serving size and protein content. For example, if a nutrition label reads "2 servings" and you plan to eat the whole package, multiply the amount of protein by 2.

Breakfast: Start The Day Off Right

When we think of breakfast protein, our minds often conjure up images of grease-laden bacon-and-sausage specials or high-cholesterol six-egg omelets dripping with melted cheese. Besides, it's so convenient to grab a bagel or a muffin when you're on the run, trying to get the kids out of the house, or racing to the office in the morning. No wonder breakfast is usually the meal people consider hardest to slip protein into and the one where they skip it altogether.

But, as you now know, leaving protein out of your morning meal sets you up to feel lethargic, light-headed, and hungry enough to start gnawing on the corner of your desk before lunch.

Believe me, I've been there. Despite everything I know about nutrition, I spent years starting my day with bowls of frosted wheat squares and milk. I still love them, but I finally came to my senses and admitted to myself that the taste wasn't worth the daily sugar crash. I feel a big difference when I choose a more balanced meal of cottage cheese with dried cranberries or my favorite oatmeal.

Can't bear to part with your bowl of O's or flakes? Why not mix a scoop of whey protein powder into the milk before you pour it over the cereal? You'll have added about 18-22 grams of protein and only about 120 more calories! (Just don't try it with chocolate-coated sugar bombs.)

Another option is to keep the cereal, but eat a source of protein like a boiled egg, Greek yogurt, or a low-fat cheese like Mini Babybel Light with it.

Here's my favorite protein-packed breakfast-on-the-go. I've made this one for professional football players as a recovery drink, too!

Jasmine's Freeze Out Smoothie

Makes 1 serving
1 cup 1% organic milk
1 cup frozen mixed berries
1 scoop natural vanilla whey protein powder
4 baby carrots
1 handful of baby spinach
Just blend and enjoy!

Time-Saving Tips

How can you fit protein into the first meal of the day when you don't have much time to whip up a high-protein omelet? It's easier than you'd think once you have a mental list of protein sources you like. (If your brain is too filled with your daily To Do list to think about menu options at 7 a.m., jot down five of your favorite breakfast protein sources and tack it to the front of your refrigerator. Your list will make it easy to remember what to shop for and what to grab in a pinch.)

Natural, nitrate-free deli ham and turkey are other protein sources I often recommend to clients for breakfast. They are both lean, high in protein, and a natural for morning because you can eat hot or cold. They are higher in sodium than some other protein sources, but you can certainly work it into the standard 2,400 mg daily sodium allowance for healthy adults. (If you have high blood pressure or other sodium-related health concerns, ask your doctor what sodium intake he or she recommends for you.) Sometimes I even wrap deli meat around a little bit of cheese for a satisfying source of protein. You can add fresh fruit for a nutritious, well-balanced breakfast that should keep you satisfied until lunchtime.

Incidentally, whenever you mix protein or fat with carbs, you lower the glycemic index (GI) of the entire meal. The glycemic index provides an estimate of how much a particular food will raise your blood sugar levels. However, since the glycemic index measures individual foods, it's important to understand that most people eat mixed meals and snacks, which alters the body's blood sugar response to the foods. (You can find out the glycemic index of most foods free of charge at GlycemicIndex.com.)

To lower your body's blood sugar response to meals, you can add protein to any number of your favorite foods. If you're a salad lover, toss in some chicken, salmon, shrimp, or even tuna. Do the same with pasta. (Be sure to make it whole wheat pasta.) Be careful not to load up your salads and pastas with hidden calorie bombs like high-fat dressings and sauces.

I love sardines. I buy them in water or lemon sauce and take them out of the can, sprinkle some lemon juice on them, and enjoy them with multi-grain crackers.

Whether you're hoping to drop a size or two, or simply to drop your old unhealthy eating habits, assessing your current protein intake and making the necessary changes is one of the most immediate and inspiring steps you can take. Talk about instant gratification. You'll see results right away in terms of how satisfied you feel and how much stamina you have.

To find new protein recipe ideas, visit the following three boards of mine:

1. Protein Recipes
2. MSF Factor Foods
3. Workout Plans.

Try it for a day or two and see for yourself! You'll be amazed by the power of protein.

Success Story: Kelly Robben

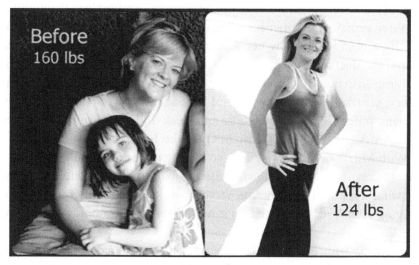

Mom of 2

first met Kelly in 2002, she was a young mom like me. Several years later, she was recovering from an injury and was unhappy with the weight she'd gained. She'd been a runner for years, so she was athletic. She decided it was time to take action, so she joined my boot camp in November 2010. She made the highest level of commitment by choosing the five-day-a-week boot camp option. To help her set and reach her goals, I evaluated her starting weight. It was higher than it should have been (160 pounds on her 5'7" frame). However, what was really shocking was her body fat—38%! While Kelly looked like she could lose some weight, her body fat was staggering. It's considered obese in terms of body fat! Like many of my clients, Kelly's unhealthy eating habits had raised her body fat levels and left her feeling both sluggish and ravenous.

I always gave my boot campers lots of nutrition information, and Kelly started following my advice to increase her protein levels, control her portions, and get better fuel for her body. She embraced my high-intensity training methods and worked hard in boot camp. In seven months, she reached her dream goal. In fact, she got beyond it—back to her high school body weight! She lost 36 pounds and reduced her body fat by 22%.

"For me, one of the biggest a-ha's was seeing that I wasn't eating enough protein," Kelly says. "That made a huge difference in my endurance, what I looked like, and feeling satisfied enough to control my portions throughout the day. Water, protein, and fiber have been my magic bullets to stop overeating."

Kelly was so inspired by her success that, though her background was in banking, she decided to become a certified trainer. Then she got certified as a boot camp instructor. Although she still does freelance work in the banking industry, her true passion is health and fitness. She started teaching for me and eventually purchased my boot camp business. Today she runs the successful Blue Valley Adventure Boot Camp in Overland Park, Kansas.

"With Mitzi's help, I stopped yo-yo dieting once and for all," she says. "She helped me realize that meeting your fitness goals isn't about endless cardio. It's about what you put in your mouth. You can work out and work out, but if you're not giving your body the nutrients it needs, you're like a hamster running on a wheel."

"Reaching your goals isn't just about transforming your clothing size and the way you look in the mirror. It's a transformation in your head, too. When you become mindful of what you put in your body, you realize that when you eat like crap, you feel like crap. Thanks to a combo of exercise and good nutrition, I feel younger today at 39 than I did 10 years ago!"

The Diabetes Epidemic

Diabetes is one of the hardest-hitting epidemics in the United States—and it's been on the rise for 20 years. It kills more Americans each year than AIDS and breast cancer combined. Most new cases are Type 2 diabetes, formerly called "adult-onset." Type 2 diabetes occurs when the body doesn't produce enough insulin, causing the body to become insulin-resistant and unable to control blood sugar levels.

Almost 26 million Americans suffer from diabetes. Another 18.8 million have it, but are undiagnosed. Another 79 million have pre-diabetes, which means their blood glucose levels are higher than normal and healthy. One in three Americans born after 2000 are at risk for developing Type 2 diabetes.

Even worse, the number of children being diagnosed with Type 2 diabetes has skyrocketed in recent decades.

In 2012, diabetes cost the U.S. an astonishing $245 billion.

The statistics are staggering—and scary.

Among the complications associated with diabetes are heart disease, eye disease, kidney disease, and nerve damage.

The best way to stave off this dangerous and potentially deadly illness is to switch to a healthy, more wholesome diet with regular exercise. Don't focus on just dropping a few pounds for the summer, but for the rest of your life. Even losing five pounds can dramatically improve blood sugar levels for people living with diabetes.

Other sounds strategies include:

- Choosing more clean foods like whole grains, lean protein, vegetables, and fruits over processed foods that are high in fat, sodium, and sugar. (MSF Factor Foods either have protein, healthy fats, or fiber/or a combination, and many of these nutrients and foods are showing great promise with blood sugar control.)
- Follow the exercise plan in chapter 11 of The Pinterest Diet (Remember to consult your physician first.)
- Educate your children about making smart, nutritious food choices and getting regular exercise.
- Visit your doctor regularly to keep tabs on your risks and to find out what you can do to lower them.

Did you know? Artificial sweeteners may be doing more than sweetening your food and drinks. A 2013 Washington University study reported in *Diabetes Care* found when obese subjects drank beverages containing sucralose (Splenda) followed by glucose, their insulin levels rose 20 percent more than subjects who drank water followed by the same amount of glucose. This suggests that artificial sweeteners could be affecting how our bodies react to glucose.

Metabolic Syndrome

Are you one of the estimated **47 million Americans** who have metabolic syndrome? Metabolic syndrome is a cluster of health conditions that increase your risk for coronary heart disease, stroke, and Type 2 diabetes. The first sign is often insulin resistance, which occurs when your muscle, liver, and fat cells are insensitive to insulin. Your body doesn't process glucose properly, so instead of taking the glucose out of your blood and moving it into your cells for energy, glucose stays in your blood and your blood sugar level remains elevated. Your pancreas continues to excrete insulin with the hopes of bringing your blood sugar down, but eventually it gets tired out.

Approximately **20 to 25 percent** of all adults in the U.S. are estimated to have this dangerous syndrome. And your chance of developing it increases if you are overweight or obese and physically inactive.

Some estimates say that one in every **10 teens**, and over **1/3** of all obese teens, also suffer from metabolic syndrome. Even more frightening, a study of **375** second- and third-graders found that **5%** had metabolic syndrome and **45%** had one or two risk factors for it. That's almost half of the lower-elementary children tested!

There are five main risk factors and many of them occur together If you have three or more of the following risk factors, you have metabolic syndrome.

1. Abdominal obesity. Excess fat in the abdominal region tends to put you at a higher risk for heart disease compared to abundant fat stored in other parts of the body, like the hips.
   Women: waist circumference equal to or greater than 35 inches
   Men: waist circumference equal to or greater than 40 inches
2. Low HDL cholesterol. HDL is categorized as the "good cholesterol" because it helps to remove cholesterol from your arteries. With low levels of HDL you are more likely to have buildup in your arteries, which raises your risk for heart disease.
   Women: less than 50 mg/dl
   Men: less than 40 mg/dl
3. High triglyceride level. When you consume more calories than you need, your body converts them into triglycerides and they may remain in your bloodstream. This can lead to a buildup of plaque in your arteries, which can cause a heart attack or stroke.
   Both women and men:
   Fasting blood triglyceride level of 150 mg/dL or greater
4. High blood pressure. When you have high blood pressure, the force of the blood against the walls of your arteries is increased, which can lead to heart damage and plaque buildup in your arteries.
   Both women and men:
   Systolic blood pressure (the top number): 130 mmHg or greater
   Diastolic blood pressure (the bottom number): 85 mmHg or greater
5. High fasting blood glucose. High fasting blood glucose may be an early sign of Type 2 diabetes, which can put you at risk for other issues such as cardiovascular disease, kidney damage, nerve damage, and more.
   Both women and men:
   100 mg/dL or greater
   To lower your risks of developing metabolic syndrome, maintain a healthy weight and aim to get 150 minutes of physical activity every week. Eat a diet with whole grains, fruits, vegetables, lean sources of protein, and healthy fats. Minimize processed foods packed with unhealthy fats, sodium, and sugar. Avoid large portions of carbohydrates.

Know Your Numbers: Make sure you ask your doctor for a blood test to check your triglycerides, HDL, and fasting blood glucose. There are some limitations of these standard blood cholesterol tests as they only identify about 40% of those at risk for coronary heart disease. I recommend a more advanced lipid testing called VAP testing, a comprehensive cholesterol test measuring 15 blood cholesterol components. It offers a far more accurate gauge of your risk of heart disease. Not all insurance companies cover it, so it might cost you $100 out of pocket. It's a test that is definitely worth the money, especially if it helps save your life! Discuss this test with your physician and I also encourage you to get your vitamin D level measured, as well.

Date	
My Triglycerides	
My HDL	
My Fasting Glucose	
My Blood Pressure	
Vitamin D	

Smart Moves For Between-Meal Munchies

Snack time gives you an ideal opportunity to pop in some protein to keep hunger at bay. You'll feel satisfied, which means you won't arrive at the lunch or dinner table famished enough to overeat and end up feeling stuffed.

The protein-rich snack options I often recommend to my clients include:

- Almonds and dried fruit
- Beef, salmon, chicken, or turkey jerky
- Boiled eggs with some fresh veggies or a piece of fruit
- Buffalo mozzarella on fresh tomatoes with basil and olive oil (one of my favorites)
- Clean energy bars (keep a pack in your desk and another in your car, or toss a few into your purse or gym bag for snack emergencies)
- Greek yogurt with chia or hemp seeds
- Natural peanut butter with a few baby carrots
- 1% cottage cheese (sweeten it up and vary the taste by mixing in some dried tart cherries or another dried fruit)

CHAPTER 7:

EATING CLEAN ON THE PINTEREST DIET

*"The food you eat can be either the safest and most powerful form
of medicine, or the slowest form of poison."*
—*Ann Wigmore*

What does it mean to eat clean? Eating clean is simply eating whole foods as close to their natural state as possible and avoiding processed and refined foods.

Why eat clean? You'll lose weight, get leaner, increase your energy levels, develop younger, healthier-looking skin, and feel better. You'll also improve your digestion and may lower your risk for heart disease, cancer, obesity, hypertension, and diabetes.

Because you'll be eating lower-calorie foods like fresh fruits and vegetables, you'll be able to eat more without gaining weight or getting bloated. And because you'll be enjoying delicious, natural flavors you'll feel more satisfied.

Despite its calorie-cutting advantages, for most people, eating clean isn't about weight loss. It's about embracing a more wholesome, healthy approach to living.

What should you eat?
1. Lean protein
2. Whole grains
3. Fresh fruits
4. Fresh vegetables
5. Healthy fats
6. Omega-3s (found in foods like salmon, sardines, walnuts)
7. Water

Choose all these foods in the purest, most unprocessed state possible. In other words, eat an orange instead of drinking orange juice. (Here's a good rule of thumb: If you can't pronounce a word in the ingredient list, don't eat the food inside the package.) Whenever possible, eat locally grown fruits and veggies when they're in season. That means they're at the peak of their ripeness, so they'll pack the most powerful nutritional punch.

Clean eating doesn't mean you have to eat raw foods, but try to use simple recipes and cooking methods. For instance, steam your broccoli; don't boil away its nutrients then smother it in sauce.

How should you eat? Follow these Pinterest Diet basics.
- Never skip a meal
- Slow down and savor each bite
- Eat smaller portions
- Stop eating when you feel satisfied

What should you avoid?
- Hydrogenated and partially hydrogenated oils (fried foods, fast foods, bakery products)

TIP: Always read the ingredient list!
- Highly processed foods
- Artificial ingredients
- Refined flour products (white rice, white pasta, white bread, white bagels, white wraps, white pita bread)

TIP: Switch to higher-fiber whole-grain versions of your favorites.
- Sodas
- Sugary fruit drinks
- Specialty high-calorie coffees
- Alcohol (especially on 7-Day Jumpstart Cleanse and then in moderation)
- Artificial sweeteners including sucralose (Splenda), aspartame (NutraSweet, Equal), acesulfame-K (Sunett), and saccharin (Sweet'N Low) TIP: some yogurts, sports drinks, diet sodas, and other zero-calorie drinks include these additives.
- Tobacco products

Mitzi's Story: Stop Smoking!

My mom died in 2003 from lung cancer. I had begged her to quit smoking for two decades. So had her doctors—and mine. I was asthmatic growing up, so I seemed to spend half my childhood in the hospital suffering from asthma attacks, pneumonia, and bronchitis. Even that didn't convince my mom to kick the habit. My mom would willingly sacrifice almost everything she could for me, but not the cigarettes.

She was diagnosed with lung cancer at the Mayo Clinic in Rochester, Minnesota, the day before she was scheduled to have a surgery to cure her newly diagnosed Cushing's Disease. I still remember leaving the building with the dreadful LUNG CANCER diagnoses ringing in my ears. It was truly my worst childhood fear coming true. I had to walk past a throng of Mayo Clinic employees who were huddled on the other side of the street where they were allowed to smoke. I could hardly stop myself from screaming at them. I wanted to ask if they really loved their cigarettes more than they loved their children and grandchildren. Instead, I ran to my car and burst into tears.

We soon learned that my mother's cancer had metastasized. She died six weeks later.

Four days after her funeral, I learned that I was pregnant with my second child.

Please don't smoke. You can rob yourself of years of life. And you can rob your grandchildren of years of happy memories with you.

Eating Clean Shopping Guide

1. Plan your menu for the week. Put everything you'll need on your grocery list, and stick to your list.
2. Never shop hungry. Temptations are harder to resist when you're ravenous.
3. Read food labels. Look for items with a short, simple list of ingredients you recognize—not unpronounceable words that sound like they belong on a chemistry exam.

TIP: Apply The 90/10 Rule

If eating clean sounds appealing, but too hard to sustain 100% of the time, try the 90/10 rule. Aim to eat clean foods 90% of the time. Leave the other 10% for dinners out, vacations, and other times when it's difficult to stick to whole, natural foods. You should still try your best to make healthful choices on these occasions. I follow the 90/10 rule myself.

"If you don't design your own life plan,
chances are you'll fall into someone else's plan.
And guess what they have planned for you? Not much."
—Jim Rohn

Slow Food: A Grassroots Twist On Health

The "slow food" movement is a cousin of the clean eating and organic food movements. Put simply, slow food is high-quality, environmentally sustainable, locally grown, natural food. (Think: heirloom tomatoes and artisanal cheese made at the farm down the road.) But the slow food philosophy is about more than *what* you eat. It involves understanding the connection between the food on your plate and the health of our planet. It's about bowing out of the fast-paced, fast-food lifestyle in favor of a more holistic approach to eating and living.

The basic principles are:
- Raising public awareness of, improving access to, and encouraging enjoyment of local, seasonal, and sustainably grown foods
- Caring for the land and protecting biodiversity for today's communities and future generations
- Conducting educational outreach in your community and to children in schools
- Identifying, promoting, and protecting fruits, vegetables, grains, animal breeds, wild foods, and cooking traditions at risk for disappearing
- Advocating for farmers and artisans who grow, produce, market, prepare, and serve wholesome food
- Promoting the celebration of food as a cornerstone of pleasure, culture, and community
  Source: SlowFoodUSA.org

I believe we should all try to live a slow food life, not only for the nutritional benefits it offers, but to support local farmers and to protect our environment. I enjoy growing my own herbs, and my daughters enjoy watching them grow. We love being able to add fresh basil from our garden to mozzarella and tomatoes in the summer. It's a great way to educate my daughters about healthy food and where it comes from.

How To Live A Slow Food Life
- Find out where your local grocery store sources their produce; buy the items that are grown locally or in your region
- Shop at local farmers' markets (To find one in your area, check out LocalHarvest.org.)
- Join a CSA (Community Supported Agriculture) program. You can find these too by checking LocalHarvest.org
- Visit local farms to educate your kids about where food comes
- Grow your own herb or vegetable garden
- Learn about food history
- Invite friends over for a dinner made from fresh, local ingredients cooked simply (Check out my Pinterest boards for tasty recipe ideas!)
- Visit SlowFoodUSAsa.org for more information. The group currently has more than 200 chapters; the website also provides information on how you can start one.

"Simplify. Be inspired. Be original. Work hard. Enjoy."
—Anonymous

Did you know? Strawberries may help to reduce inflammation. A 2011 study by researchers at UC Davis found that overweight adults who consumed the equivalent of about ⅔ cup of strawberries in a beverage daily had lower levels of inflammation and insulin resistance after eating a meal with a moderate level of fat. It's no surprise that The American Diabetes Association identifies berries as one of the top 10 super foods for diabetics. They're packed with vitamins, antioxidants, and dietary fiber—and strawberries seem to help the insulin in our bodies work more effectively.

Furthermore, a 2012 Harvard study showed that eating two or more servings of strawberries a week delayed cognitive aging in women by up to 2.5 years. So, something as simple as boosting your berry intake could boost your brain health!

Inflammation And Foods To Fight It

You now know that eating clean can improve your health. Did you know that it can help combat inflammation, too?

The word "inflammation" is thrown around in nutrition circles a lot lately. The term actually refers to the body's natural response to infection and injury. It's an important defense mechanism that helps our body to heal by bringing nutrients and immune cells to the affected area.

> **Did you know? Tart cherries have the highest anti-inflammatory content of any food. Check out my Chocolate-Covered Cherry Smoothie recipe to help reduce chronic inflammation!**

Chronic inflammation, on the other hand, is damaging. It leads to a host of problems, from the painful swelling associated with arthritis to diabetes to heart disease to cancer. There are four keys to reducing chronic inflammation:

1) eating a healthy diet
2) getting regular exercise
3) reducing stress
4) weight management

Clean foods also happen to be highly effective anti-inflammatory foods. They include:

1) **Foods high in omega-3s.** Great sources include salmon, herring, mackerel, sardines, anchovies, trout, flaxseeds, and walnuts. FYI: An imbalance of omega-6 and omega-3 fatty acids can trigger inflammation, and the average American diet includes 10 times more omega-6 fatty acids (those found in nuts, seeds, and vegetable oils) than omega-3s.

2) **Extra virgin olive oil.** Olive oil contains a natural anti-inflammatory agent that may contribute to low levels of heart disease among people who adhere to a Mediterranean diet.

3) **Antioxidant-rich foods.** These include non-citrus fruits and vegetables. The more colors you eat, the better. Each color corresponds to a different health-promoting phytochemical. Some good choices to eat regularly are strawberries, blueberries, raspberries, papaya, cantaloupe, apricots, cherries, plums, and watermelon. Antioxidant-rich vegetables include

kale, carrots, spinach, broccoli, cauliflower, squash, pumpkin, bell peppers, sweet potato, and turnip greens.

4) **Spices.** Fresh ginger, garlic, and rosemary. You can also check your pantry for cinnamon, coriander, and turmeric. They're all great choices to use in cooking. If you have a high-powered blender or juicer, start the day with a green smoothie that combines fresh ginger, leafy greens like kale or spinach, and any fruits you like. Apple, baby carrots, and ginger make for a great combination as well. (Check out my smoothie recipes in this book and my Pinterest boards for more delicious smoothie recipes!)

Thirsty? Green tea contains phytochemicals that help fight inflammation and promote joint health. Studies suggest you'll need to drink 3 to 4 cups a day to see the benefits. Enjoy a steaming mug in the winter or cool off by making your own refreshing iced version in the summer!

CHAPTER 8:

THE PINTEREST DIET 7-DAY JUMPSTART CLEANSE

"Without passion life is nothing."
—Anonymous

Don't worry! The Jumpstart program in this chapter is NOT an extreme "cleanse" like the ones that have become so popular with celebrities in recent years. It's a simple, well-balanced, protein-rich, weeklong eating plan designed to energize you, accelerate your weight loss, and eliminate the bloat and fatigue that unhealthy highly processed foods can trigger. My Jumpstart plan emphasizes lean proteins, fresh fruits and vegetables, fiber, and healthy fats.

Worried about your sweet tooth? Missing wine with dinner? Rest assured, this is the only indulgence-free week on *The Pinterest Diet.* You can treat yourself to your favorite Planned Indulgences in the weeks that follow.

But before we get started, I want to weigh in on juice-only cleanses.

WARNING: As a registered dietitian and nutritionist with 17 years of professional experience, I would NEVER advise a liquid cleanse. Why? It can be downright dangerous to your health! Most liquid cleanses are usually extremely low—or completely lacking—in protein. They put a strain on your body in lots of ways when you go on them for several days or weeks.

Cleanses are harmful to:

- Your muscles: Since the majority of cleanses force you to give up solid food and restrict you to drinking juice, your body takes in mostly sugar on a cleanse. That makes your insulin levels spike and crash, which can leave you shaky, dizzy, and nauseous. You're also apt to have trouble concentrating.

Without real food, your body doesn't get all the calories it needs, so you start to use up your protein stores and lose muscle mass. Once you start eating regular foods again, you'll have less muscle to burn calories—and the calories will be more likely to turn into fat. Odds are, you'll regain all the weight you lost . . . and probably a few pounds more.

- Your brain: After several days on a low-protein cleanse, your brain's neurotransmitters stop functioning effectively. You'll start to feel fuzzy, unfocused, irritable, and depressed.

- Your kidneys: The proteins in your muscles start to break down after a few days on a liquid cleanse, which means chemicals start to run into your bloodstream. Your kidneys have to work extra hard to detoxify your blood.

- Your intestines: Due to lack of activity, the villi (little finger-like formations that line your small intestine and help your body absorb the nutrients in food) start to atrophy. This can cause diarrhea, which leads to dehydration.

The verdict? While cleanses might help you lose weight in the short term because they're so ultra-low in calories, it's a temporary fix. In the long run, cleansing is likely to do your body more harm than good. You've got to start eating solid food again sooner or later—and when you do, if you're like most people, you'll gain back every pound you lost. Probably more. It's yo-yo dieting at its worst.

The solution?

The best way to lose weight and keep it off is by eating a "clean" diet 90% of the time. Focus on fresh, wholesome foods like whole grains, fruits, veggies, legumes, fish, nuts, and lean meats. Avoid highly processed packaged foods that are loaded with trans fats, sugars, and preservatives. Liquid cleanses won't counteract the effects of an unhealthy diet. They'll just add to the damage you're doing to your body.

So, forget juice cleanses forever. Instead, try the easy-to-follow, nutrient-packed Pinterest Diet alternative below.

Mitzi's 7-Day Jumpstart Cleanse

7-Day JumpStart Cleanse Rules:

1. No alcohol, coffee, or soft drinks. Drink only water and green tea. Remember to take your weight in pounds and divide by 2 to get the minimum number of ounces of water you should be drinking daily. (For instance, if you weigh 140 pounds, try to drink 70 ounces of water.) You can replace soda with sparkling water. My favorite is LaCroix, a 100% natural sparkling water that is calorie-, sweetener-, and sodium-free.

TIP: Can't live without caffeine? If you're a coffee drinker, cut your daily intake by 50% for the first 2 days. Then eliminate it altogether for the rest of the week.

2. Absolutely no eating after 7:30 p.m. This will be KEY to your success!

3. No snacking. Eat three meals a day or two meals plus one smoothie.

4. Choose one of the Jumpstart options for breakfast, lunch, and dinner every day. Portion sizes might need to be adjusted based on your current weight. They are based on a diet for a female who weighs about 140 pounds.

5. Record your daily food intake as discussed in chapter 4.

6. Eat a source of protein at every meal to keep yourself feeling satisfied. To make it easy for you, all the breakfasts I've included in this chapter contain 15 to 25 grams of protein. The lunches and dinners all include at least 30 grams of protein.

7. Take a daily high-quality fish oil supplement.

7 Breakfast Options

Choose your favorites throughout the week. If you repeat a few meals, that's fine.

1. ¾ cup of rolled oats mixed with ½ cup 1% organic milk (no packaged oatmeal). It only takes 90 seconds to make in the microwave. Sprinkle cinnamon and 3 sliced strawberries on top with 2 teaspoons of sliced almonds. Add 2 to 3 more tablespoons of 1% organic milk.
2. ½ cup 1% cottage cheese + 1 cup watermelon
3. 2 eggs scrambled with baby spinach + apple
4. 1 cup non-fat Greek yogurt with 1 teaspoon honey + orange
5. Jasmine's Freeze Out Smoothie:
   1 cup 1% organic milk
   1 cup mixed frozen berries
   large handful of baby spinach
   4 baby carrots
   1 scoop natural vanilla whey protein powder
6. Chocolate-Covered Cherry Smoothie
   1 cup 1% organic milk
   1 cup frozen tart cherries
   1 scoop natural chocolate whey protein powder
7. Pure Banana Smoothie
   1 cup 1% organic milk
   1 frozen banana
   1 scoop natural vanilla whey protein powder

7 Lunch Options

Choose your favorites throughout the week. If you repeat a few meals, that's fine.

1. 4 to 6 oz. grilled chicken breast on 3 cups romaine, 10 green grapes, 5 toasted walnuts, 1 tablespoon crumbled gorgonzola cheese; 2 tablespoons balsamic vinegar as dressing
2. 4 to 6 oz. tuna on 3 cups baby spinach with 1 sliced Granny Smith apple; 2 tablespoons balsamic vinegar as dressing
3. Small whole wheat tortilla, ¾ cup black beans, ½ oz. shredded cheese, dollop of light sour cream, salsa; 1 cup berries
4. 2 oz. sliced buffalo mozzarella, 2 whole tomatoes sliced, balsamic vinegar, 1 teaspoon extra virgin olive oil; 1 cup melon
5. 1 whole wheat sandwich thin with 1 tablespoon natural peanut butter, 1 tablespoon honey, medium sliced banana
6. 1 can of sardines in lemon sauce with 18 Special K Multi-Grain Crackers; 8 strawberries
7. 4 to 6 oz. grilled chicken stuffed into ½ whole wheat pita, 2 tablespoons hummus, ¼ cup chopped tomatoes, 1 tablespoon crumbled feta; 1 apple

7 Dinner Options

Choose your favorites throughout the week. If you repeat a few meals, that's fine.

1. 5 to 6 oz. grilled salmon; ½ cup brown rice; 8 baby carrots; 1 cup fruit of your choice
2. 5 to 6 oz. lean ground beef, ¾ cup whole wheat spaghetti pasta with ½ cup marinara sauce; 3 cups baby spinach with cherry tomatoes, and 3 sliced baby carrots; balsamic vinegar as dressing; 1 cup watermelon
3. 1 cup Avocado Chicken Salad (see chapter 10) on whole wheat sandwich thin;1 cup of berries of your choice
4. 5 to 6 oz. grilled chicken; ½ cup cooked wild rice; 4 asparagus spears; 1 peach
5. 5 to 6 oz. Spice Rubbed Pork Tenderloin (see chapter 10); Baked Sweet Potato (see chapter 10); 1 banana
6. 2 hard shell tacos with 3 oz. lean ground beef in each with sliced lettuce and tomato, 1 tablespoon mozzarella cheese and 1 teaspoon light sour cream on each, top with salsa; 1 kiwifruit
7. 4 to 6 oz. nitrate-free deli meat of your choice on whole wheat sandwich thin with Laughing Cow Light cheese wedge and 2 teaspoons Dijon mustard; 8 strawberries

Pinterest Pointer:

Don't forget to consult my Pinterest boards this week. I'll have some great MSF Factor-Approved Smoothies pinned, as well as updates and helpful hints to use during your 7-Day Jumpstart Cleanse.

You'll be starting your 7-Day Jumpstart Cleanse at the same time you start *The Pinterest Diet* Workout. That means you'll be eating less and exercising more. That first week will be the toughest, but do your best. If you haven't worked out in years, it'll be a big adjustment at first. Hang in there! Both the meal plan and the fitness plan are designed to give you a safe, well-balanced introduction to losing weight and improving your health. If you're struggling and need motivation, just log on to Pinterest and spend some time re-energizing yourself by reading your Daily Inspiration Board!

"Your life is your message to the world. Make sure it's inspiring."
—Anonymous

CHAPTER 9:

THE PINTEREST DIET PROGRAM

"The way you think, the way you behave, the way you eat,
can influence your life by 30 to 50 years.
—Deepak Chopra

F ollowing The Pinterest Diet, you will . . .

1.   Stop making excuses and start living a healthier lifestyle today
2.   Use Pinterest for a never-ending supply of delicious recipes and workout plans
3.   Use Pinterest as your ultimate dream board to create the body and life you want
4.   Customize your food intake to match your Unique Taste DNA
5.   Learn how to eat to keep yourself satisfied and avoid mindless munching
6.   Lose weight and create the healthy new habits you need to keep it off for good in just 30 days

Taking 100% Responsibility, Taking Charge

Let's set the record straight: You are your current weight, size, and shape—whether you admit it or not—because of the choices you've made. Stop the excuses. No one forced you to eat the bag of chips at midnight; you chose to eat it. You chose whether or not to exercise yesterday. Many of us get used to blaming, justifying, or complaining instead of taking full responsibility for our own lives. We blame our spouse, kids, parents, boss, friends, lack of time, lack of money, and anything else we can find for our problems. It's convenient. And it makes us feel less guilty. But it prevents us from reaching our health and fitness goals—and often our life goals.

If you want to transform your body, make a vow never to blame, justify, or complain again. It might be challenging at first. But, as you'll soon discover, it's a life-changing step. It's the key that will enable you to live a healthier, happier life.

Admit to yourself:

I chose sugary soda instead of water.

I rarely went to the gym.

I ate when I wasn't hungry.

I drank too much alcohol.

I ate portions I knew were too big.

> **TIP:** One of my favorite ways to get people to be aware of how much they complain is by gifting them with a Complaint Free World bracelet, founded by Kansas City pastor, Will Bowen. They can be purchased at AComplaintFreeWorld. org. Pastor Bowen has appeared on Oprah and The Today Show and to date has provided over 10 million bracelets worldwide. Each time you complain you must switch the wrist you wear your bracelet on and you need to go 21 consecutive days without complaining in order to "graduate" from the program. It is a very powerful tool that helps people become more aware of their complaining ways. I have even passed them out to a group of Major League Baseball players while I was speaking to them at Spring Training.

Now that you've accepted 100% responsibility for where your life is right now, assure yourself that it's okay. Everybody makes mistakes. Don't dwell on what you've done wrong. You're not a bad person. You're not weak. But you're not going to keep making those mistakes.

To succeed at losing weight (or reaching any goal, for that matter), you need to think in positive, success-oriented terms. That means ending the blame game—whether you've been using external factors as an excuse not to lose weight or beating yourself up for your lack of self discipline. Odds are, every one of those negative thoughts is a simple misperception that you're hanging onto for no reason. Any time you catch yourself with self-defeating thoughts ("I had fried food for lunch, so I blew it. I'll never lose this weight!" "Dieting has never worked for me before, so why should it this time?") . . .

STOP!

Take a deep breath.

Now reprogram that negative self-talk into a more positive, promising message. Believe it or not, if you change your expectations about what will happen, you can actually change the outcome for yourself! You can go from pessimism to optimism. Here's an example: Say, you slip up and eat a whole order of greasy French fries for lunch after following *The Pinterest Diet* program perfectly for a week. If your reaction is negative (you chastise yourself for falling off the weight-loss wagon, you fume at your friend for tempting you into ordering the fries in the first place, you convince yourself that all your hard work was useless), you'll probably give up and fail. But if you change your reaction (put a more positive spin on it by saying, "So what? It's one meal; it's not the end of the world. I'll do better at most of my other meals."), you'll up your odds of success enormously.

It's not easy to reprogram your internal voice from "I can't" to "I can," but keep practicing. It takes time to overcome old habits and replace them with more productive new ones.

Here's a helpful hint: Next time you feel like giving up, go to your Daily Inspiration Board, read the motivational quotes and look at photos of the kind of body you want. Look at the beach vacation spot where you want to wear your bikini and feel fabulous. Now, close your eyes, relax, breathe slowly, and try to visualize yourself happy and confident at your goal weight. Make the vision as specific as possible. What are you wearing? Where are you? Who are you with? What are you doing? What's the weather like? Indulge your imagination and enjoy the fantasy. The more time you spend thinking about it and the more detailed you make the vision, the more real it's likely to seem. As the old saying goes, if you can dream it, you can do it. And *The Pinterest Diet* provides you with the ultimate dream board.

Don't forget to Pin 10! Keep updating your Pinterest boards daily with images that remind you of your goal—great outfits you want to buy, activities you'd like to try, a vacation you'd like to take when you reach your target weight. In addition to collecting new pins, spend time perusing the pins you've already collected to remind yourself to stay focused on the happy ending rather than obsessing over the struggle to get there.

Keep in mind that you have the power to:

Choose water.

Go to the gym.

Avoid non-hunger-inspired eating.

Limit alcohol intake.

Stop eating when you feel satisfied.

You *can* do it!

> *"Healing is a matter of time, but it is sometimes*
> *also a matter of opportunity."*
> —Hippocrates

Set Your Goals

Success books have touted the importance of setting goals for years. (Hey, if you're going to reach them, you've got to set them first!) And the crucial first step of setting any goal is to put it on paper. Seeing your goals in writing makes them real. In fact, research shows that the simple act of writing down a goal makes you more likely to achieve it. Listing your health and fitness goals is just as important as writing down anything else you want to achieve in life.

I want you to set concrete, specific weight loss goals and turn them from simple wishes and longings to actionable items you can really achieve. (Instead of "I want to lose weight", you'll decide, "I will weigh 130 pounds by May 31, 2014.") Incidentally, you can use these principles for any goal, whether it's financial, career-related, or even romantic.

First, I want you to write down three goals. Go to my website (NutritionExpert.com) to download a handy goal sheet to use. Once you've filled out the sheet, look at your goals at the beginning of every day and again at the end of the day. Reviewing them twice *every day* is one of the keys to making them reality.

Once you've set your goals, sign your name to show you've made a commitment to reach them. Next, **TAKE ACTION**! Don't wait a minute longer. Take your first step now toward creating your own life as you want it to be.

Five Strategies For Success:
1. Find the Time

Start paying attention to the time-wasters in your life. Maybe it's an hour of television. Perhaps it's an hour you spend typing social emails at the end of every workday. Resolve to use the time more productively—by going to the gym, doing a burpee Tabata, or making a healthy, home-cooked meal. Sometimes these are easy to give up. Sometimes they require a bit more self-sacrifice. But the result will be worth the effort.

2. Stop The Clean Plate Syndrome

An astonishing 54% of adults report they clean their plate every time they eat. Many of us were conditioned to do this as kids. Remember all those starving children in other parts of the world? They were many a mom's favorite incentive for forcing you to keep shoveling food in until every morsel disappeared. Result: Years later, we're still inhaling it all like human garbage disposals regardless of how full we're feeling. In fact, many of us don't even *realize* how full we're getting as we're eating. We use the clean plate as the litmus test to tell us that we're satisfied rather than tuning in to our own bodies' hunger and satiety cues.

Why do we still clean our plates as adults? Countless reasons. Habit. Reluctance to waste good food. The echoes of our parents' voices whispering in our ears to "clean our plate." Cost. ("I paid for it, I'm going to finish it—especially if it's a restaurant meal.") Getting rid of all the food in front of us gives us a sense of satisfaction. ("Hey, I completed a task—even if it *was* just polishing off an enormous bowl of spaghetti.") We're focusing on something other than eating (conversation, a television show, a magazine article). Or, simply: It tastes good.

It's time to start listening to your body and honoring it. That's prerequisite number one for getting the bod you dream of.

So, forget all those old childhood rules. I *am* giving you permission to *leave food on your plate.* In fact, I'm encouraging it. You should never again clean your plate. If someone you're eating with gets offended that you didn't clean your plate, blame it on me. Tell them, "My nutritionist told me to always leave some food on my plate!" Typically, the more food you leave, the better. Even if you're making your own meals and serving yourself small portions, leave a little on your plate. Why? It's the first step in taking charge of your eating—you're going to teach yourself to control it instead of letting it control you.

Skeptical? Believe me, it works—even for professional athletes. And they have some of the biggest appetites anywhere! I introduced the no-more-clean-plates concept to an All-Star Major Leaguer who used it as his main strategy to get leaner. During Opening Day for the Royals, I was sitting with his wife, and she told me how amazed she'd been to see her husband leaving food on his plate at every meal—something she'd never seen him do before. This simple solution helped him shed 16 pounds and feel much better. If it worked for him, it can work for you!

Once you get the hang of leaving food behind, you can start tuning in to your hunger cues more effectively. You'll also start to eat more slowly and take more pleasure in eating, recognizing when you're getting satisfied, and stopping before you're stuffed.

Sure, it takes some getting used to. Old habits die hard. But you'll be amazed at how much power you'll feel when you push your plate away and decide that you've eaten enough to satisfy yourself. If you're struggling, repeat after me: Those last few bites are better in the Hefty bag than on my belly or my butt.

I know my approach works because I've used it myself. After years of struggling with my own weight despite all I knew about nutrition and fitness, I got my best body at 33—after having two kids, no less—by following the same program I help my clients learn to apply to their daily lives. I've got more energy and I feel healthier and happier with my body than ever!

3. Cure Calorie Amnesia

One of the first steps toward successful weight loss is getting over what I call calorie amnesia. It's the self-deluding belief that nothing you ate while standing over the kitchen sink "counts." Same goes for the tidbits you ate while rummaging through the refrigerator looking for a snack or while preparing your children's lunches for school. Stop kidding yourself! Strive for conscious eating. Remember, you should always sit down at the kitchen table or the dining room table when you eat in your home—and savor your food slowly.

4. Enjoy Planned Indulgences

See if this sounds familiar: You baked cookies. Okay, so maybe you bought them. There are only five left. You eat them all, figuring "Better get rid of them so I won't be tempted tomorrow when I start my diet." Here's another scenario: You go out to dinner and gorge on everything from appetizers to sides to dessert. You even eat the mint that comes with the bill. Might as well enjoy it now; the diet starts first thing in the morning.

You just had "The Last Supper."

The problem occurs when you have four "Last Suppers" a month! You're always planning to start your diet the next day or the next month or after you eat everything in the kitchen.

Oddly enough, we often use dieting to justify overeating. We develop an all-or-nothing, feast-or-famine thinking. You know the pendulum will swing back the other way . . . eventually. So putting yourself on a strict diet where you swear off all the guilty pleasures you love sets you up to fail every time. As I said earlier, restrictive eating leads to overeating. Always has, always will.

You might find this a surprising confession from a nutritionist, but I keep chocolate in my house at all times. I don't leave cookies sitting out on the counter because I know that sooner or later in a moment of weakness or a fit of the munchies, I'll walk in and grab a handful even if I'm not hungry. (Been there, done that.) I put really good, healthy snacks like a bowl of fresh fruit out in plain sight, so my family and I will grab those instead. But I also buy bite-size chocolate caramel candy. When the occasional chocolate craving strikes, I don't gnaw my fingernails for hours trying to fight it or force down a rice cake as a placebo. I eat chocolate.

It's time to start making smart choices. That means taking control of what you eat, but it doesn't mean being overly restrictive. You're not trying to punish yourself. You're trying to nurture yourself. Instead of obsessing over the foods you think you *shouldn't* eat, you need to reprogram your thoughts to focus on the foods you *should* eat for good health, such as the MSF Factor Foods while also including Planned Indulgences.

Learn how to negotiate so that you'll be able to enjoy all the foods you love without overindulging or omitting the nutrients you need for good health. For example, if you look forward to enjoying a glass of wine with dinner every night, you can do it, but you need to cut back elsewhere. You might cut down on your bread or rice. Meeting a friend for dinner at the restaurant that serves the best mud pie in town? You might agree in advance to share an entrée to leave yourself more calories for dessert.

By the way, if you're like my clients, you're probably assuming I eat healthy, low-fat, low-cal foods all the time. Not so. I'm a foodie. I *love* to eat. I also love sweet indulgences. If you don't believe me, check out my Sweet Indulgences Board on Pinterest. I don't make these recipes on a regular basis and I don't want you to either, but they're fine to enjoy on occasion. Whenever I go to a restaurant, I scan the menu for the dish that sounds most delicious. That's what I order. If it turns out to be the most nutritious, great. If not . . . *I still order it.* (Granted, I try to pick restaurants that offer fresh, seasonal ingredients whenever possible.) Naturally, I'll adjust my other meals, my exercise levels, and my portion size to make it work for me, but I'm not going to deprive myself of what I want.

As I tell my clients, don't fight the foods you love—work with them. That's the one and only way you'll lose weight for good and make sensible, healthy eating a permanent part of your lifestyle.

5. Be Bold

Try something you've never tried before at least once a week. Sample new flavors and enjoy whole foods in their natural state. It's amazing how delicious simple foods can taste. I hope *The Pinterest Diet* will help you discover a whole new world of exciting food and mouthwatering recipes. Remember, I'm no Martha Stewart in the kitchen, and I don't expect you to be one either. Food doesn't have to be complicated or time-consuming to be tasty and good for you!

Little Things Add Up To Big Results

I wish I could say you'd wake up thinner tomorrow after reading this chapter. But unfortunately, the weight you've spent years putting on won't melt away by eating well and exercising for one or two days. Losing weight takes effort, day after day, week after week, and month after month. I do know that if you follow my program outlined in this book you can transform your life in 30 days.

Persistence always pays off. Problem is, it's not so easy to persevere. And it's very easy *not to*. If you're not careful, one or two days of skipping your workout will turn into one or two weeks, then one or two months and before you know it, it's time to make your New Year's Resolution to lose weight *again*!

Just remember . . .

Successful people do what unsuccessful people aren't willing to do.

Pin this message on your Daily Inspiration Board. You might also want to write it down and tape it to your fridge, your bathroom mirror, your computer, your dashboard—wherever you need inspiration. Keep it in your mind on the days when you'd rather skip exercising or clean your plate even if you know it's loaded up with twice as much food as you need.

Keep in mind, too, that little things make a BIG difference over time. Small, daily personal choices can make or break your success. And you get results by taking baby steps every day, like leaving a little bit of food on your plate, even if it's only one or two bites. The next day, leave a little more. The same goes for exercise: Get to the gym or do a four-minute workout in your living room. Do it today, tomorrow, and the next day. Even if you devote 10 minutes, four times per week to working out in your house, you *will* see a difference. Do it until you feel worse on the days when you don't exercise than on the days when you do. By that point, you'll *want* to hit the gym or don those workout shoes to do burpees and mountain climbers! The key is to consistently do the small things that will add up to major results.

Before you know it, you'll feel more energetic, be more productive, and look better! You won't reach your ultimate goal in seven days, but you *will* start feeling better in that time frame and see results. You *can* see major results in 30 days when you keep it up and stay focused.

Business and organization experts sometimes call this "the Swiss cheese" method of tackling projects: You punch little holes in the big project one by one—small, manageable, bite-sized "holes"—so that you don't get overwhelmed and give up in despair. Keep the big picture (yourself happy and healthy and looking fantastic at your goal weight) in mind, but approach the process patiently, a day at a time, congratulating yourself for even the smallest positive changes.

And make sure you Pin 10 every day!

At first, you'll probably feel uncomfortable leaving food on your plate. You'll probably feel awkward exercising, too, if you haven't worked out in a while—or ever. You will probably feel sore. But if you stick with it, that will soon change. I know you can do it!

Your goal is to feel uncomfortable on the days you are *not* practicing the principles of *The Pinterest Diet*. Don't worry; you'll get there. Just focus on doing a few little things on a daily basis—a better food choice here, more activity there—and they'll become much easier to do!

> *"Either you run the day or the day runs you."*
> —*Jim Rohn*

Journal It!

I highly recommend that you write down what you eat every day in a food log. (Go to PinterestDiet.com to download your free food log.) Do it after every meal or once a day—whatever works for you. It's not designed to make you fess up to "cheating." It's simply the best way to find out whether you're eating the foods that will make you feel most satisfied—the ones that will allow you to listen to your body's natural hunger and satiety cues and to eat fewer total calories without going hungry. Plus, you'll be able to figure out what you're doing right and where you're struggling, whether it's with a certain meal or time of day or whether there are certain foods you're overlooking and others you're focusing on too much.

You don't have to count any calories on *The Pinterest Diet*. But to give you a snapshot of how important it is to eat the right foods and avoid the wrong ones, here's a quick calculation: One pound of fat = 3,500 calories. That means, to drop a single pound on the scale, you'd need to eat 500 fewer calories for seven days in a row or burn 500 extra calories every day for a week or—my favorite—combine eating less with moving more! You get the idea.

12 Foods You MUST** TRY on The Pinterest Diet	
1.	Chia seeds
2.	Clif Kit's Organic Bar
3.	Freekeh
4.	Kale
5.	Kefir
6.	Hemp seeds
7.	LaCroix Water
8.	Sardines
9.	Seaweed
10.	Simply Snackin Jerky
11.	Quinoa
12.	Teff
** Make an exception to this rule if you have allergies to any of the foods above.	

Foods You Should Eat On The Pinterest Diet

In chapter four, I shared my 50 Top MSF Factor Foods with you. The list below includes many of those foods too (they're noted with an *), but it also includes foods that are antioxidant powerhouses and some that just barely missed the top 50. They might not quite qualify as MSFs because they're not rich enough in healthy fats, protein, or fiber. However, they're still full of nutrition.

Fruits		
Apples*	Goji berries	Papaya
Apricots	Grapefruit	Peaches
Avocados*	Grapes	Pears*
Bananas*	Guava	Persimmons
Blackberries*	Honeydew	Pineapples
Blueberries*	Kiwifruit*	Pomegranates
Cantaloupe	Limes	Plums
Cherries*	Lemons	Raisins
Coconut	Mangoes	Raspberries*
Cranberries	Nectarines	Strawberries*
Dates	Oranges	Watermelon*
Figs	Prunes*	

Vegetables

Acorn squash	Eggplant	Radishes
Artichokes	Fennel	Rainbow chard
Arugula	Garlic	Red onions
Asparagus	Ginger, fresh	Romaine lettuce
Beets	Green beans	Rutabagas
Bell peppers	Horseradish	Shallots
Bok choy	Jicama	Snow Peas
Broccoli	Kale*	Spinach*
Brussels sprouts	Leeks	Squash
Butternut squash	Lettuce	Sweet potatoes*
Cabbage*	Mushrooms	Swiss chard
Carrots*	Okra	Tomatoes
Cauliflower	Onions	Turnips
Celery	Parsnips	Turnip greens
Collard greens	Peas	Watercress
Corn	Peppers (hot: cayenne, chili jalapeno)	Water chestnuts
Cucumbers	Peppers (sweet: red, orange, green, red)	Yellow squash
Dandelion greens	Pumpkin	Zucchini
Endive	Radicchio	

Grains

Amaranth*	Couscous (whole wheat)	Quinoa*
Barley*	Duram	Spelt
Buckwheat	Freekeh*	Teff
Brown rice	Kamut*	Wheatberries
Bulgur	Millet	Wheat bran
Chia seeds*	Oats* (old-fashioned rolled oats and steel-cut)	Whole wheat bread, pasta, pita, English muffins, etc.*
Corn tortillas	Oat bran	Wild rice

Beans and Legumes*

Adzuki beans	Great Northern beans	Navy beans
Black beans	Green peas	Split peas
Black-eyed peas	Kidney beans	White beans (cannelloni or Northern)
Butter Beans	Lentils (brown, green, red)	
Garbanzo beans (chickpeas)	Lima beans	

Nuts, Seeds, and Nut Butters

Almond butter*	Hazelnuts	Pumpkin seeds
Almonds*	Hempseeds	Sesame butter
Brazil nuts	Macadamia nuts	Sesame seeds
Cashew butter*	Peanut butter*	Sunflower seeds
Cashews	Peanuts*	Tahini
Chia seeds*	Pecans*	Walnuts*
Flaxseeds	Pine nuts	Other nut and seed butters made from above list (natural only)
Hempseeds, hulled	Pistachios*	

Dairy

Cheeses, natural*	Cottage cheese, 1%*	Low-fat plain yogurt
Cream cheese, reduced fat	Kefir	Organic milk, 1%*
Chocolate milk, 1%	Low-fat organic Greek Yogurt*	Sour cream, light

Soy Products

Edamame (soybeans)	Natto
Fermented soy products (tempeh and miso)	Tofu (limit to twice monthly)

Eggs

Organic, cage-free, omega-3 eggs*

Fats and Oils

Almond oil	Flaxseed oil	Pumpkin seed oil
Avocado oil	Hemp seed oil	Sesame oil (unrefined, cold pressed, organic)
Coconut oil*	Macadamia nut oil	Walnut oil
Extra virgin olive oil* (do not use for sautéing as it has a low smoke point)	Olive Oil	

Fish and Seafood

Barramundi	Mackerel*	Sardines*
Clams*	Mahi Mahi	Scallops*
Cod*	Mussels*	Shrimp*
Crayfish*	Oysters*	Tilapia, US
Lobster	Salmon, wild*	Tuna*

Meat and Poultry		
Bison	Lamb	Pork tenderloin*
Chicken breasts, skinless*	Lean ground beef such as Laura's Lean Beef*	Turkey breasts
Filet mignon	Pork chop	Venison

Beverages (including non-dairy milks)		
Almond milk	Fresh vegetable and fruit juices	Rice milk
Coffee	Hemp milk	Tea (green, black, white, and yerba mate)
Cranberry juice	Pomegranate juice	Wine (preferably red)

Sweeteners
Honey

Herbs, Spices, and Condiments		
Use any fresh and dried herbs and spices. Some of the best ones are listed below.		
Apple cider vinegar	Cumin	Parsley
Balsamic vinegar	Garlic	Pepper
Barbecue sauce	Ginger	Rosemary
Basil	Horseradish	Sage
Black pepper	Hot sauce	Salsa
Broths, organic, low-sodium (vegetable and chicken)	Ketchup	Sea salt
Cardamom	Light mayo	Soy sauce (low-sodium)
Cloves	Mustard	Thyme
Cinnamon	Oregano	Turmeric

Other
Chocolate, dark (at least 70% cocoa)

Did you know? Cranberries truly do reduce your risk of getting a urinary tract infection (UTI). They have anti-adhesion properties, which prevent bacteria from adhering to the lining of your urinary tract. That's especially good news now that some viral infections and the E. coli bacteria that cause UTIs are becoming increasingly resistant to commonly prescribed antibiotics. Research suggests that drinking cranberry juice cocktail regularly helps to reduce the risk of getting a UTI.

The Pinterest Diet Plan

To help you focus on the foods you need for good nutrition instead of focusing on those you *shouldn't* eat, use the following guidelines. I use them for all my clients as a formula for successful weight loss.

- Eat three **MSF Factor Foods** every day.
- After calculating your individual **protein** needs in chapter six, aim for 15 to 30 grams of protein for breakfast and a minimum of 30 grams for lunch and dinner.
- Eat a source of **fiber** and protein at every meal to help you stay satisfied.
- Eat at least one source of **omega-3s four days each week**.
- Aim to eat at least one source of **healthy fat** every day.
- Aim to completely eliminate trans fats from your diet. Read food labels carefully. Limiting fast food and avoiding commercially baked goods will be your best bet for getting trans fats out of your diet.
- Use **fruits and vegetables** to "expand your plate" each day. It really helps to satisfy.
- Eat 1½ to 2 cups of **fruit** per day.
- Eat 2 to 2 ½ cups of **vegetables** a day.
- Eat 4-6 servings of **whole grains** a day. To accelerate your weight loss, choose a portion in the lower part of the range. Carbs aren't bad for you, but most of us eat too many of them. An easy rule of thumb: **ONE serving** of whole grains has about 15 grams of carbs.
- Drink plenty of **water**. Remember, drink ½ your weight in ounces!
- Take a daily **fish oil** supplement.
- Take a daily **multivitamin** with **minerals** that includes **vitamin D**.

The Pinterest Diet Menu

Variety might be the spice of life, but studies show that people are more likely to succeed at projects like losing weight when they have a plan that minimizes the number of decisions they have to make. So I encourage you to simplify your life by picking your top one to two choices and eat them regularly.

You can also look back at the Jumpstart Breakfast Options in chapter 8 for additional ideas. (*means recipe is available in Chapter 10)

The Pinterest Diet Breakfast Options

1. ¾ cup cottage cheese, 1 slice whole wheat toast, 1 cup strawberries
2. Banana Chocolate Smoothie*
3. Kiwi Strawberry Smoothie*
4. Blue Banana Chocolate Smoothie*
5. Mitzi's Oatmeal*
6. 6 oz. non-fat Greek yogurt, 1 cup mixed berries
7. 2 eggs scrambled, 1 cup fruit, 6 oz. Greek yogurt

Pick three or four meals you like best from the list below, and eat them regularly to make lunchtime easy and satisfying. You can also look back at the Jumpstart Lunch Options in chapter 8 for additional ideas or later in this chapter at the 14-Day Pinterest Diet Meal Plan.

The Pinterest Diet Lunch Options

1. 4 to 6 oz. grilled chicken, 1 whole wheat sandwich thin, 8 baby carrots, 1 banana
2. 4 to 6 oz. tuna or chicken salad, 1 whole wheat sandwich thin, 8 strawberries
3. 4 to 6 oz. tuna or grilled chicken, 2 cups baby spinach, 1 tablespoon of walnuts, 1 oz. feta cheese, and balsamic vinegar as dressing, 15 grapes
4. ¾ cup whole wheat tortilla, black beans, ½ oz. shredded cheese, dollop of light sour cream, salsa, kiwifruit

5. 1½ cups Mitzi's Quick and Clean Chili*, 4 whole wheat crackers, 1 peach or pear
6. 4 to 6 oz. egg, or chicken salad on 2 cups baby spinach, 1 tablespoon walnuts, with 1 sliced Granny Smith apple, balsamic vinegar/olive oil dressing (3 parts balsamic vinegar; 1 part oil)
7. Bowl of miso soup, sashimi/sushi (2 pieces tuna, 2 pieces eel, 2 pieces salmon, 2 pieces yellowtail), 1 cup mixed berries
8. 1 can of sardines in water or lemon sauce with 18 Special K Multi-Grain Crackers; 8 strawberries
   See The Pinterest Diet Recipes for additional options.

Unlike breakfast and lunch, it's a good idea to vary your dinners regularly so you won't get bored. You can also look back at the Jumpstart Dinner Options in chapter 8 for additional ideas or later in this chapter at the 14-Day Pinterest Diet Meal Plan. For dinner, you may pick a Planned Indulgence from the list provided in this chapter.

The Pinterest Diet Dinner Options

1. 5 to 7 oz. salmon, ¾ cup quinoa or brown rice, 1 cup baby carrots
2. 5 to 7 oz. grilled chicken breast, ¾ cup beans, 1 cup cooked spinach
3. 5 to 7 oz. pork tenderloin, 1 whole wheat sandwich thin, 2 cups mixed greens with balsamic vinegar
4. 5 to 7 oz. grilled shrimp, ¾ cup whole wheat linguini, ½ cup marinara sauce, 1 cup carrots and tomatoes
5. 5 oz. grilled chicken, ½ whole wheat bun, 1 sliced tomato, and 1 oz. mozzarella
6. 5 to 7 oz. filet mignon or ground bison, whole wheat roll or bun, 1 cup asparagus
7. 5 to 7 oz. grilled chicken in whole wheat tortilla with black beans, light sour cream, salsa, 2 cups mixed greens with balsamic vinegar with 5 toasted pecans
8. 5 to 7 oz. pork chop, baked sweet potato, 2 cups salad greens with balsamic vinegar
9. 5 to 7 oz. fish such as salmon, ¾ cup whole wheat pasta, ½ cup marinara sauce, 1 cup broccoli

MSF Factor Snacks
- 49 pistachios
- 23 almonds
- 10 baby carrots with hummus
- Clif Kit's Organic Bar
- 1 orange
- 1 apple
- 1 cup strawberries
- 1 medium banana
- 1 cup fresh pineapple
- 2 cups watermelon
- 1 cup low-fat or nonfat Greek yogurt
- 2 oz. beef, salmon, venison or turkey jerky
- ½ tuna sandwich
- 1 hardboiled egg
- 2 oz. sardines with Special K Multi-Grain Crackers
- 0.2 oz seaweed snack
- ½ cup 1% cottage cheese
- 1 Mini Babybel Light cheese wedge between 2 Special K Multi-Grain Crackers
- Peanut butter, honey and banana on whole wheat sandwich thin
- Handful of raw nuts or seeds and dried fruit
- 3 slices fresh buffalo mozzarella and tomato with basil, balsamic vinegar, and drip of olive oil
- ½ cup 1% cottage cheese with fruit or 6 whole wheat crackers
- ½ of ham, tuna, turkey, roast beef, sandwich with raw veggies
- ½ whole wheat pita with tuna salad or hummus
- 1 cup low-fat plain yogurt with 1 tablespoon ground flaxseed and fresh fruit
- Banana with 1 tablespoon peanut butter or other nut butter
- Apple with 1 tablespoon peanut butter or other nut butter
- ¾ cup black beans with salsa and light sour cream
- 1 cup berries with 1 cup 1% milk
- ¾ cup Avocado Chicken Salad*
- 1 Mini Babybel Light with 8 strawberries
- 1 hardboiled egg
- ¾ cup tuna or chicken salad on ½ whole wheat sandwich thin

- 2 cups popcorn (unbuttered)
- ¾ cup of 6 Bean Salad*
- ½ peanut butter and jelly sandwich
- ¼ cup guacamole and 10 black bean or sweet potato chips
- ½ cup cottage cheese with ½ cup salsa and 10 black bean or sweet potato chips

Drink Choices:
- Water (with lemon or lime if desired)
- Green tea
- Wine (one glass, optional at dinner—and only after you complete the 7-Day Jumpstart Cleanse)

Did you know? A U.S. review conducted by the *Journal of Agricultural and Food Chemistry* found that eating a diet rich in berries can reduce the ageing process and improve brain health. Scientists believe the antioxidants and phytochemicals in berries protect the brain from oxidative stress produced by free radicals. The study also found the berries had anti-inflammatory properties, which prevented neuronal damage and improved both cognitive and motor functioning.

Planned Indulgences:
- Eat juicy fruit approximately every other day with dinner as your Planned Indulgence: 1 cup fresh berries/melon/fruit.
- You don't have to eat your Planned Indulgence at dinner. You can eat it earlier in the day but do not eat it any later than 7:30 pm.
- On the days you're not eating your favorite fruits alone (about every other day) as your Planned Indulgence, you can enjoy one of the following:

  - 1 oz. dark chocolate (made with at least 70% cocoa)
  - Peach Crumble*
  - Frozen Greek Yogurt Banana Pops*
  - Greek Yogurt-Covered California Strawberries*
  - Peanut Butter Honey Greek Yogurt Dip* with fresh fruit
  - Frozen Banana Peanut Butter Bites*
  - Honey Peanut Butter Protein Energy Balls*

- Skinny "Fried" Honey Bananas*
- Strawberry Watermelon Lemonade*
- Skinny Prosecco*
- Hot cocoa (use skim milk)
- Skinny Strawberry Sangria*

As mentioned previously, you can still enjoy your favorite piece of carrot cake on occasion. Just make sure you adjust the rest of your diet and exercise plan accordingly.

Making The Plan Work For You

As you know by now, *The Pinterest Diet* is all about eating what's right for YOU. It's not generic. It's designed to be tailored to your Unique Taste DNA and your goals. The following sample daily diet plans are designed simply to give you a framework for your meals. Feel free to switch meals around, to ignore those that don't appeal to you, and to repeat those you love. Then again, if you want to take the brainwork out of deciding what to eat, follow the plan exactly.

Always remember to stop eating when you feel satisfied and to eat more of the foods that help to make you feel most satisfied. The bottom line is to lose weight you need to eat less than what you ate to reach your current weight. So, use smaller bowls and plates, eat less of everything than you used to, and savor every bite.

Eating Your Favorite Foods On The Pinterest Diet

As promised, *The Pinterest Diet* allows you to include the foods you LOVE. Not all the time, though. And not in any amount, of course. If you did the worksheets in chapter five, you've compiled a list of your all-time top 10 favorite not-so-healthy foods—the ones that appeal most powerfully to your Unique Taste DNA. Depending on how quickly or slowly you want to reach your weight loss goals, you can plan to include them in your diet once a month or once a week. Just make sure you keep the portions in check. You can nibble on your favorites more frequently if you keep the portions even smaller. Simply substitute a small, single-portion size of your favorite food into the appropriate category, whether it's a dessert, protein entrée, whole grain, salad, etc.

My Personal Favorites:
- Chicken Madeira with asparagus and rye bread from The Cheesecake Factory (I eat it about once every three weeks and share *one* portion with my husband and two daughters.)

- Chocolate molten lava cake with vanilla bean ice cream (I share this once every few months with my family.)
- Ben & Jerry's Chunky Monkey (I eat this about every 3 to 4 months)

Remember: There's no need to overindulge in your favorites now that you KNOW you'll be able to have them again soon. Maybe not tomorrow, but before long *you will get to eat them again*. Amazingly, people often find that once they've gotten used to eating healthier they no longer love certain "bad" foods as much. Sometimes they find their old standbys leave them sluggish and bloated. You get to decide on this one, though. I'm trusting you to use common sense.

14-Day Pinterest Diet Meal Plan

Day 1
Breakfast: Strawberry Baked Oatmeal Casserole*
Lunch: 6-Bean Salad* + Kale Chips* + Kiwifruit
Afternoon Snack: ½ cup 1% cottage cheese with 10 dried cranberries
Dinner: Grilled Salmon* + Parmesan Roasted Asparagus*
Planned Indulgence: 1½ cups watermelon and cantaloupe
Drinks: Water (with lemon/lime), green tea

> TIP: Try LaCroix sparkling water for a delicious flavor without artificial ingredients.

Day 2
Breakfast: Leftovers from the Strawberry Baked Oatmeal Casserole*
Lunch: Mitzi's Quick and Clean Chili* + apple
Afternoon Snack: ¼ cup Slow Cooker Honey and Cinnamon Nuts*
Dinner: ¾ cup cooked whole wheat spaghetti with ¾ cup of marinara sauce with 96% lean ground beef
Planned Indulgence: Skinny "Fried" Honey Bananas*
Drinks: Water (with lemon/lime), green tea

Day 3

Breakfast: Mitzi's Oatmeal*
Lunch: Balela Salad* + Lemon Parmesan Kale Salad* + 15 grapes
Afternoon Snack: ½ whole wheat pita with 2 oz. tuna + 2 teaspoons non-fat Greek Yogurt
Dinner: Taco Pizza*
Planned Indulgence: 1 peach + ½ cup raspberries
Drinks: Water (with lemon/lime), green tea

Day 4

Breakfast: Straw-Banana Smoothie*
Lunch: ¾ cup black beans + 1 oz. mozzarella cheese + dollop of light sour cream + salsa (heat black beans and cheese in microwave for 30-40 seconds) + 8 strawberries
Afternoon Snack: 10 dried tart cherries with 10 almonds
Dinner: Balsamic Chicken in the Slow Cooker* + ¾ cup brown rice + Steamed Spinach*
Planned Indulgence: 1 oz. dark chocolate (made with at least 70% cocoa)
Drinks: Water (with lemon/lime), green tea

Day 5

Breakfast: Honey Quinoa Breakfast Bake*
Lunch: Pistachio Cranberry Freekeh Salad*
Afternoon Snack: Honey Cinnamon Roasted Chickpeas*
Dinner: Honey Pecan Salmon* + Parmesan Roasted Asparagus*
Planned Indulgence: 8 strawberries + Peanut Butter Honey Greek Yogurt Dip*
Drinks: Water (with lemon/lime), green tea

Day 6

Breakfast: Kiwi Strawberry Smoothie*
Lunch: Leftover Pistachio Cranberry Freekeh Salad*
Afternoon Snack: ½ cup salsa + ½ cup 1% cottage cheese + 10 black bean chips (mix together salsa and cottage cheese to dip chips into)
Dinner: Spice Rubbed Pork Tenderloin* + Balsamic Baby Carrots*
Planned Indulgence: Peach Crumble*
Drinks: Water (with lemon/lime), green tea

Day 7

Breakfast: Mitzi's Oatmeal*
Lunch: Caprese Salad* + Watermelon Feta Salad*
Afternoon Snack: 1 container of sardines packed in lemon sauce + 8 whole wheat crackers
Dinner: Lime Avocado Chicken* + Skinny Six Layer Dip* + 8 black bean chips
Planned Indulgence: Greek Yogurt Covered California Strawberries*
Drinks: Water (with lemon/lime), green tea

Day 8

Breakfast: Jasmine's Freeze Out Smoothie*
Lunch: Your choice; Pick your favorite!
Afternoon Snack: Mini Babybel Light with 15 grapes
Dinner: Grilled Salmon* + Sweet Potato Casserole*
Planned Indulgence: 1 oz. dark chocolate (made with at least 70% cocoa)
Drinks: Water (with lemon/lime), green tea

Day 9

Breakfast: Honey Quinoa Breakfast Bake
Lunch: 2 cups baby spinach + 5 oz. grilled chicken + 1 tablespoon crumbled Gorgonzola + 2 tablespoons balsamic vinegar + 1 cup berries
Afternoon Snack: Simply Snackin Jerky Treat
Dinner: 96% Lean Laura's Lean Beef hamburger + ¼ avocado + 2 slices tomato on whole wheat sandwich thin
Planned Indulgence: Hot cocoa
Drinks: Water (with lemon/lime), green tea

Day 10

Breakfast: 6 oz. non-fat Greek yogurt + banana
Lunch: ½ whole wheat sandwich thin with 2 slices fresh mozzarella on top: Melt 30 seconds in microwave, top with 2 slices tomato + ¼ of avocado + 2 tablespoons balsamic vinegar
Afternoon Snack: Clif Kit's Organic Bar-Berry Almond

Dinner: Skinny Caprese Roll-Ups*
Planned Indulgence: ½ cup light vanilla ice cream + 1 cup berries
Drinks: Water (with lemon/lime), green tea

Day 11

Breakfast: Banana Chocolate Smoothie*
Lunch: 4 oz. nitrate free deli turkey on whole wheat sandwich thin +
1 tablespoon mustard and 1 Laughing Cow Light cheese wedge
+ 15 grapes
Afternoon Snack: Honey Peanut Butter Protein Energy Balls*
Dinner: Whole wheat Tortellini and Shrimp Salad*
Planned Indulgence: Strawberry Salsa* + Whole Wheat Cinnamon
Crisps*
Drinks: Water (with lemon/lime), green tea

Day 12

Breakfast: Strawberry Baked Oatmeal Casserole*
Lunch: 1 tablespoon peanut butter + 2 teaspoons honey + sliced
banana on whole wheat sandwich thin
Afternoon Snack: Mini Chocolate Covered Cherry Smoothie*
(divide ingredients in half)
Dinner: Grilled Salmon* + Kale Chips* + Watermelon Feta Salad*
Planned Indulgence: Hot cocoa
Drinks: Water (with lemon/lime), green tea

Day 13

Breakfast: Mitzi's Oatmeal*
Lunch: Avocado Chicken Salad* + 1 apple
Afternoon Snack: Honey Cinnamon Roasted Chickpeas*
Dinner: Quick and Easy Spinach Lasagna* + Mitzi's Strawberry
Salad
Planned Indulgence: Frozen Greek Yogurt Banana Pops*
Drinks: Water (with lemon/lime), green tea

Day 14

Breakfast: Blue Banana Smoothie*

Lunch: Caprese Grilled Cheese* + Lemon Parmesan Kale Salad* + 1 cup mixed fruit

Afternoon Snack: 1 container of sardines packed in lemon sauce + 8 Special K Multi-Grain Crackers

Dinner: Spice Rubbed Pork Tenderloin* + Baked Sweet Potato*

Planned Indulgence: 1 oz. dark chocolate (made with at least 70% cocoa)

Drinks: Water (with lemon/lime), green tea

* Recipe included in *The Pinterest Diet Recipes*

On Your Mark! Get Set! Go!

Now you have all the information you need. So, don't wait until tomorrow or the first of next month. Get on your way to the body and the weight you've dreamed about *now*!

To Cheat Or Not To Cheat?

This book is about creating an entirely new lifestyle. The good news is that once you get used to *The Pinterest Diet*, you'll feel so much better that you'll want to stick to it. But that doesn't mean you have to give up cake forever! I want you to enjoy your life. So, go ahead and have a slice of cake on your birthday. Or at your favorite restaurant that happens to serve the best cheesecake on the planet. Remember, on *The Pinterest Diet*, we call these Planned Indulgences. One of my absolute favorite guilty pleasures is molten lava cake with a scoop of vanilla bean ice cream. I still enjoy it once every few months and try to get someone to share it with me. Afterward, I don't feel guilty. I just start eating well again.

Remember, restrictive eating leads to overeating. It would be unrealistic for me to order you to give up your favorite indulgence foods permanently. Are you really going to swear off French fries for the rest of your life? However, if you're like most of my clients, you may be surprised to discover that your tastes change as you grow accustomed to a healthier way of eating. Some of the old indulgence foods you once deemed irresistible might not taste as appealing anymore. This is especially common if you start eating clean.

The most important success strategy I can share with you is to stick with it. Little improvements add up over time and lead to positive results. Just make sure you don't let a day of bad eating turn into a week, a month, or a year of it. Never give up! Lifestyle changes require a shift not just in your behavior but in your mindset. You're embracing a new way of thinking about yourself, your future, and how you feed and care for your body. So, forgive yourself when you slip up, but value yourself enough to get right back on track!

CHAPTER 10:

THE PINTEREST DIET RECIPES

"You can't out-exercise a bad diet."
—Anonymous

Mitzi's Cooking Philosophy
I didn't grow up dining out at fancy restaurants. In fact, I didn't even try sushi until I was 24! Like most mothers at that time in America, my mom made the majority of our meals from scratch, but I also remember dipping potato chips in Miracle Whip. Whoa! That's a fat-drenched snack I hope my kids will *never* try—or even know about unless they read this book!

These days, smart choices are the number one rule in my kitchen. But I approach cooking like I approach the TV interviews I do: I keep it simple. If I can get fabulous flavor with three to four ingredients, I don't bother using eight.

If you lack confidence in the kitchen, you're not alone. Lots of people do. Stop worrying! You don't have to be Martha Stewart to make a delicious dish. All the recipes in this chapter are easy enough for the most confirmed cooking-phobe to follow. And remember, even if a recipe calls for six ingredients, if you can make it tasty using only three, feel free to scrap the others.

Kitchen Basics: Building Your Pinterest Diet Kitchen
Make sure you've got these kitchen staples on hand to cook the recipes in *The Pinterest Diet.*
- Blender
- Cutting boards
- Nonstick skillet
- BPA-free plastic containers with lids for leftovers
- Set of knives

- George Foreman Grill and/or outdoor grill
- Baking dishes
- Measuring cups and spoons
- Stockpot
- Mixing bowls
- Rubber spatulas
- Nonstick cooking spray (my faves are coconut oil and olive oil sprays)

Mitzi's Modifications: 10 Ways To Make Recipes Healthier

One of my absolute favorite things to do is to find recipes featuring food that fits my Unique Taste DNA and tweak them to improve both their nutritional value and their flavor. Working with recipes is so much fun for me and one of my favorite parts of writing this book!

Look for my repins of recipes with Mitzi's Modifications.

Here are 10 of my favorite tricks for making recipes healthier.

1. Switch all pasta, rice, bread, and tortillas from white to whole wheat. When refined grains are processed, they lose the germ and bran, which contain about 90% of the grain's nutrients. Whole-grain products retain the germ and bran, which means they're packed with nutrients and help to prevent several chronic diseases.

2. Switch from corn, soy, sunflower, and canola oil to olive oil, almond oil, avocado oil, coconut oil, macadamia nut oil, walnut oil, or extra-virgin olive oil. Recipes often call for more oil than you really need, so reduce it to decrease your calorie intake.

A Word About Oils

I have five favorite oils. I use them all frequently in cooking.

Coconut oil. is wonderful to cook with because it has a high smoke point of 450°F. Also, as I mentioned earlier, the saturated fat in coconut oil is the healthier kind, with MCTs. Buy virgin or extra virgin coconut oil. It's never hydrogenated or partially hydrogenated, which makes it healthier for you.

Extra virgin olive oil. is another oil I love. It's great for salads and dishes that don't need to cook at high heat because it has a lower smoke point. Avoid using it for recipes that require oven temperatures above 350°F.

My other top picks are almond oil, macadamia nut oil, and olive oil.

---

3. Instead of using mayonnaise in sandwiches, wraps, and dips, use avocado, hummus, Greek yogurt, mustard, or light mayo. Mayonnaise is high in fat, calories, and sodium. The other options are packed with healthy fats and protein.

4. Use lean meat products like poultry without the skin and lean cuts of beef, pork, and lamb instead of high-fat ones for meals. Lean meat sources contain less saturated fat and won't increase your cholesterol like high-fat meats. Pick ground meats that are between 94% and 96% lean and contain less than three grams of fat per ounce.

5. Use honey instead of white or brown sugar in baking. Both honey and sugar contain glucose and fructose, but all-natural honey is sweeter and denser, so you won't have to use as much in recipes when baking.

6. Add vegetables to every meal to make it healthier and more filling. Vegetables are loaded with nutrients and antioxidants, but are low in calories. Toss them into whole wheat pasta dishes, salads, sandwiches, wraps, casseroles, smoothies, or just eat them on their own.

7. Decrease or eliminate butter in recipes. I do use butter when I make cookies and love it on a piece of bread when I go to a restaurant, but it's high in calories and saturated fat. I know it's tasty, but try cutting back on the amount of butter in recipes. Butter is often loaded onto foods like vegetables and casseroles, which is not necessary.

8. Choose low-sodium canned beans and tomatoes. Low-sodium chicken, beef, and vegetable broth and low-sodium soups tend to be healthier choices. Also, drain and rinse your beans. You'll reduce the sodium content by about 40%.

9. Replace salt in recipes with natural herbs and spices. You'll preserve the flavor and reduce your sodium intake, which helps decrease the risks of serious chronic diseases associated with high sodium intake. To add a boost of flavor to your recipes, try pepper, garlic powder, celery seed, chili powder, paprika, dill, or rosemary. (For more ideas, check out the section about spices in this chapter.) You often can eliminate the salt in recipes without making them taste any less delicious, so don't stress about finding the perfect herb or spice replacement. If you need to follow a low-sodium diet you must check out my favorite source for amazingly delicious low sodium recipes, *Sodium Girl's Limitless Low-Sodium Cookbook*. Sodium Girl also has wonderful recipes on Pinterest at Pinterest.com/SodiumGirl.

10. Choose 1% organic milk, almond, or hemp alternatives instead of high-fat dairy products. High-fat dairy products are loaded with calories and they contain a significant amount of saturated fats, which can be dangerous in large quantities. 1% organic milk contains 10 grams of protein per cup. Hemp and almond milk options are plant based and higher in healthy fats. They're also a good choice for anyone who can't tolerate dairy products.

"Always do your best. What you plant now, you will harvest later."
—*Og Mandino*

SMOOTHIES

Smoothie Tips And Tricks

Minis: You can make mini versions of any of my smoothies by dividing all the ingredients in half.

Bananas: The secret to making frozen bananas for smoothie add-ins is to peel ripe bananas and place them immediately in a resealable freezer bag. Bonus: Frozen bananas make great snacks for kids, too.

Building the best smoothie: It doesn't have to be an architectural masterpiece, but there is a little art to making a tasty smoothie. Put the larger, harder, chunkier ingredients like frozen fruits in the blender first, like frozen bananas. They'll be closer to the blade, which ensures that they'll be adequately chopped up. Next add large, soft, solid ingredients like seeds, cottage cheese, and leafy greens. Powders come next, and, finally, liquids. If you're using ice, put it in either first or last but never between layers of ingredients.

SMOOTHIE ADD-INS

Almonds	Fish oil	Mangoes
Avocado	Flax seed	Matcha
Baby carrots	Garlic	Mint
Bananas	Ginger	Nutmeg
Beets	Goji berries	Oats
Blueberries	Goji powder	Parsley
Chard	Grapes	Peanut butter
Cherries	Greek yogurt	Protein powder (whey, hemp)
Chia seeds	Green tea	Pumpkin seeds
Cinnamon	Hemp seeds	Spinach
Cloves	Honey	Spirulina
Cocoa powder	Kale	Strawberries
Coconut flakes	Kefir	Swiss chard
Coconut oil	Lemon	Watermelon
1% cottage cheese	Limes	Wheat germ
Cucumbers	Maca powder	Wheat grass

*"Optimism is the faith that leads to achievement.
Nothing can be done without hope and confidence."*
—Helen Keller

141

Smoothies

Banana Chocolate Smoothie

Makes 1 serving

1 cup 1% organic milk
½ frozen banana
1 scoop natural chocolate whey protein powder

Just blend and enjoy!

Blue Banana Chocolate Smoothie

Makes 1 serving

1 cup 1% organic milk
½ frozen banana
½ cup fresh blueberries
1 scoop natural vanilla whey protein powder

Just blend and enjoy!

Chocolate-Covered Cherry Smoothie

Makes 1 serving

1 cup frozen tart cherries
1 cup 1% organic milk
1 scoop natural chocolate whey protein powder

Just blend and enjoy!

Jasmine's Freeze Out Smoothie

Makes 1 serving

1 cup 1% organic milk
1 cup frozen mixed berries
1 scoop natural vanilla whey protein powder
4 baby carrots
1 handful of baby spinach

Just blend and enjoy!

Kiwi Strawberry Smoothie

Makes 1 serving

1 cup 1% organic milk
½ frozen banana
1 cup California strawberries
1 kiwifruit (peeled)
1 scoop natural vanilla whey protein powder

Just blend and enjoy!

Straw-Banana Smoothie

Makes 1 serving

4 large California strawberries
½ banana
1 cup 1% organic milk

Just blend and enjoy!

Breakfast Dishes

Mitzi's Oatmeal

Makes 1 serving

¾ cup old-fashioned oats
1¼ cup 1% organic milk
1 teaspoon cinnamon
2 teaspoons brown sugar or honey

Put the oats and ¾ cup milk in the microwave for 1 minute 30 seconds. Let sit for 15 seconds. Then add up to another ½ cup milk. Sprinkle with cinnamon and brown sugar or honey. Optional: I often add fresh strawberries and 2 teaspoons of sliced almonds to give the oatmeal more nutritional punch and to make it more satisfying.

Honey Quinoa Breakfast Bake

Makes 9 servings

1 cup quinoa (uncooked)
1 tablespoon cinnamon
2 cups mixed frozen berries
2 organic eggs
2 cups 1% organic milk
¼ cup honey
½ cup coarsely chopped nuts

Preheat oven to 350°F. Spray an 8x8 baking dish with nonstick cooking spray. In a small bowl, stir together the uncooked quinoa and the cinnamon, making sure the quinoa is well coated. Pour quinoa over bottom of prepared dish. Spread the berries and nuts evenly over the top of the quinoa. In a small bowl, lightly beat the eggs. Add the milk and honey to the beaten eggs and whisk together. Pour the egg mixture on top of the quinoa and berries. Bake 1 hour or until the breakfast bake only has a small amount of liquid remaining. Serve warm.

Recipe created by Mitzi. Reprinted with permission from National Honey Board.

Strawberry Baked Oatmeal Casserole

Makes 9 servings

2 cups old-fashioned oats
⅓ cup brown sugar
1 teaspoon baking powder
1 ½ teaspoons cinnamon
¼ cup chocolate chips
½ cup walnut pieces
1 ½ cups sliced California strawberries
2 cups organic 1% milk
1 large organic egg
1 teaspoon vanilla extract
1 banana

Preheat oven to 375°F. Spray a 9x13 baking dish with nonstick cooking spray. In a large bowl, mix together oats, sugar, baking powder, cinnamon, 2 tablespoons of the chocolate chips, half of the walnuts, and half the berries. In another large bowl, mix together the 1% organic milk, egg, and vanilla extract. Now, add the oat mixture to the baking dish. Add the remaining berries, chocolate chips, and walnuts. Top with a layer of bananas. Slowly pour the milk mixture over the oat mixture and shake gently to coat evenly. Bake 30 to 40 minutes, until top is golden brown and milk is set.

Lunch Dishes

Avocado Chicken Salad

Makes 2 servings

2 (5 oz.) cooked chicken breasts, torn apart
½ avocado, diced
2 tablespoons non-fat plain Greek yogurt

Gently mix all ingredients together. Eat alone or on top of one side of sandwich thin.

Balela Salad (Middle Eastern Bean Salad)

Makes 6 serving

1 can (15 oz.) chickpeas, drained and rinsed
1 can (15 oz.) black beans, drained and rinsed
1 cup tomatoes, chopped
½ cup green onion, chopped
1 garlic clove, minced
2 tablespoons extra virgin olive oil
2 tablespoons lemon juice
¼ cup cider vinegar
½ cup fresh parsley, chopped
Sea salt, to taste
Black pepper, to taste

Gently mix all ingredients together. Chill and serve.

Caprese Grilled Cheese

Makes 1 serving

2 slices of whole wheat sandwich bread
2 oz. fresh mozzarella, sliced into rounds
1 Roma tomato, sliced

1 tablespoon basil, chopped in ribbons

Spray a nonstick skillet with nonstick cooking spray. Heat to medium. Place mozzarella on the bread and top with tomato and basil. Once the bread is slightly brown, flip the sandwich carefully and cover with lid. Cook until golden brown and cheese is melted through. Serve immediately.

Caprese Salad

Makes 1 serving

2 oz. fresh mozzarella, sliced
1 tomato, sliced
¼ avocado, sliced
2 tablespoons balsamic vinegar
2 tablespoons fresh basil
Sea salt, to taste

Layer ingredients. Variation: Chop all ingredients and toss them together gently.

Quick and Clean Chili

Makes 5 servings

14 oz. 96% lean ground beef
1 onion, chopped
2 cloves garlic, minced
1 (14½ oz.) can of low sodium tomatoes, cut up (can also used diced canned tomatoes)
2 (15 oz.) can dark red kidney beans, drained and rinsed
1 (8 oz.) can tomato sauce
1 tablespoon chili powder
¼ cup fresh basil, chopped

In a large stockpot, cook lean ground beef, onion, and garlic. Once meat is brown, drain fat. Add undrained tomatoes, kidney beans, tomato sauce, chili powder, and basil. Bring to a boil. Reduce heat, cover, and simmer for 20 to 25 minutes.

Appetizers & Snacks

Honey Cinnamon Roasted Chickpeas

Makes 4 servings

1 can (15.5 oz.) Great Value chickpeas
1 teaspoon olive oil
1 tablespoon honey
½ teaspoon cinnamon
pinch of salt

Preheat oven to 375°F. Drain and rinse chickpeas, towel dry. Spread evenly on baking sheet lined with foil. Bake for 30 to 40 minutes, until crunchy. Mix honey, oil, cinnamon, and salt until well blended. Remove chickpeas from oven and toss with honey mixture to coat. Return the coated chickpeas to the baking sheet, spreading them out evenly in a single layer, and bake for 5 to 10 more minutes to caramelize, taking care not to burn.

Recipe created by Mitzi. Reprinted with permission from Wal-Mart Stores, Inc. © 2013 Wal-Mart Stores, Inc.

Honey Peanut Butter Protein Energy Balls

These are a great pre- or post-workout option.
Makes 2 dozen

1¼ cup old-fashioned oats
3 tablespoons shredded coconut
½ cup sliced almonds, chopped
1 tablespoon hemp seeds, shelled (optional)
1 scoop whey protein powder
½ cup honey
½ cup dried apricots, chopped
½ cup peanut butter

In a medium bowl, combine the oats, coconut, almonds, hemp seeds and protein powder. Stir until well distributed. Add the honey, apricots, and peanut butter, and stir all ingredients well. Put mixing bowl into the refrigerator for 20 to 30 minutes. Then roll into rounded balls. Chill. Will last refrigerated for about 5 days.

Recipe created by Mitzi. Reprinted with permission from National Honey Board.

Skinny Six-Layer Dip

This is a great make-ahead appetizer for a party or tailgating.
Makes 16 servings

1 can (16 oz.) non-fat refried beans
1 cup part-skim mozzarella cheese
1 cup cheddar cheese
1 (8 oz.) container light sour cream
1 cup guacamole
1 cup salsa

In a 9 x 13 inch glass baking dish, spread the refried beans on the bottom. Sprinkle ½ the mozzarella and cheddar cheese on top of the beans. Spread sour cream evenly over cheese. Add the guacamole, then the salsa. Top with the remaining cheese. Serve with black bean tortilla chips. Serve at room temperature or refrigerate to chill.

Slow Cooker Honey and Cinnamon Nuts

Makes 4 servings
1 (⅓ cup each) cup raw almonds, walnuts, and pecans
½ teaspoon cinnamon
2 tablespoons honey

In a medium bowl, combine nuts and cinnamon. Add honey, and stir to coat nuts. Add to slow cooker, cover, and cook on low for 1 hour. Let cool before serving.

Strawberry Salsa

Makes 6 servings

2 cups California strawberries, hulled and finely chopped
2 kiwifruits, peeled and finely chopped
2 tablespoons lime juice
2 tablespoons fresh cilantro

In a medium bowl, gently mix together all ingredients. Serve on top of grilled chicken or fish. Or serve with baked whole wheat cinnamon chips (see recipe).

Whole Wheat Cinnamon Crisps

Makes 4 servings

2 whole wheat pitas
1 teaspoon Cinnamon
1 teaspoon Sugar

Preheat oven to 350°F. Spray a large baking sheet with non-fat cooking spray. Cut pita in half, then into wedges with a pizza cutter. Mix cinnamon and sugar together. Sprinkle both sides lightly with cinnamon sugar mixture. Bake 10 minutes or until crisp.

Entrees

Balsamic Chicken in Slow Cooker

Makes 3 serving

1 lb. chicken breasts2 cans (15 oz.) low-sodium diced tomatoes
½ cup balsamic vinegar1 tablespoon garlic, minced
Pepper, to taste
Sea salt, to taste

Place all ingredients in slow cooker on low heat. Cook for 6 to 8 hours on medium or 4 to 5 hours on high.

Grilled Salmon

Makes 4 servings

4 (5 oz.) salmon fillets
1 tablespoon olive oil
Juice of a lemon
Sea salt, to taste

Heat grill to medium-high. Meanwhile, brush salmon with oil. Brush grill grate with oil. Place salmon, skin side down, on grill and cover. Cook about 10 to 15 minutes, until the fish flakes easily. Allow 10 additional minutes for each extra inch of thickness. Remove from grill and top with lemon juice and sea salt.

Honey Pecan Salmon

Makes 3 serving

¼ cup of whole wheat panko breadcrumbs
¼ chopped pecans
2 tablespoons + 1 teaspoon of honey
2 tablespoons mustard
3 (5 oz.) salmon fillets

Preheat oven to 425°F. Mix breadcrumbs, pecans, honey, and mustard. Spread the chunky mixture evenly over the top of the salmon fillets. Put the salmon in the oven for 10 to 12 minutes, or until the topping is golden brown.

Recipe created by Mitzi. Reprinted with permission from National Honey Board.

Lime Avocado Grilled Chicken

Makes 4 servings

4 (5 oz.) boneless chicken breasts
juice from a lime
1 avocado, peeled and cut into chunks
1 teaspoon extra virgin olive oil
2 tablespoons fresh cilantro, chopped

Grill chicken on medium heat. Gently mix together the lime juice, avocado, olive oil, and cilantro. Top each chicken breast with the avocado mixture.

Quick and Easy Spinach Lasagna

Makes 9 servings

8 oz. package whole wheat lasagna noodles (9 strips)
25 oz. prepared spaghetti sauce
32 oz. organic non-fat or 1% cottage cheese
6 oz. mozzarella cheese, shredded
6 oz. cheddar cheese, shredded
6 oz. fresh baby spinach

Preheat oven to 350°F. In a 9x13 baking pan, place a small amount of spaghetti sauce to coat the bottom. Place three strips of uncooked lasagna noodles in the pan lengthwise. Spread with ⅓ of the spaghetti sauce, ⅓ of the cottage cheese, ⅓ of the spinach, ⅓ of the mozzarella, and ⅓ of the cheddar cheese. Repeat the layering process two more times. Cover with nonstick foil and bake for 30 minutes, then remove foil and continue baking an additional 30 minutes. Let stand 10 minutes.

Six-Bean Salad

Makes 15 servings

1 can (15 oz.) low-sodium dark red kidney beans, drained and rinsed
1 can (15 oz.) low-sodium black beans, drained and rinsed
1 can (15 oz.) butter beans, drained and rinsed
1 can (15 oz.) black beans, drained and rinsed
1 can (15 oz.) northern white beans, drained and rinsed
1 can (15 oz.) garbanzo beans (chickpeas), drained and rinsed
1 medium onion, diced
½ cup carrots, shredded
¾ cup red wine vinegar
3 tablespoons extra virgin olive oil
¼ cup sugar

Combine the drained and rinsed beans in a large bowl. Add onion and carrots. Separately, whisk together the red wine vinegar, extra virgin olive oil, and sugar. Pour over bean mixture. Refrigerate at least 2 hours before serving to allow flavors to develop.

Skinny Caprese Roll-Ups

Make 8 servings

8 whole wheat lasagna noodles, uncooked
¾ cup Great Value part skim ricotta cheese
1 large Great Value organic egg white
⅓ cup Great Value finely shredded Parmesan cheese
14 oz. freshly shredded, Great Value low-moisture part skim Mozzarella cheese
4 medium Roma tomatoes, thinly sliced (about 1/6 inch thick)
1/4 cup chopped fresh basil, plus more for garnish
1¾ cups light marinara sauce

Preheat oven to 350°F. Cook pasta according to package directions. Drain, but do not rinse with water. Place lasagna noodles in a single layer on a large sheet of wax paper. In a mixing bowl, whisk together ricotta cheese and egg white until well blended. Stir in Parmesan cheese. Add 12 oz. mozzarella cheese. Evenly spread ¼ cup of the cheese mixture over each lasagna noodle. Place the sliced tomatoes over the cheese mixture. Sprinkle fresh basil on top. Tightly roll each of the lasagna noodles. Spread about ⅓ cup marinara sauce in the bottom of a 9 x 12 baking dish. Place the lasagna roll-ups seam side down in the dish. Top each roll-up with about 3 tablespoons of marinara sauce, making sure to cover the edges so they won't dry out while baking. Sprinkle the top with the remaining 2 oz. shredded mozzarella. Bake 30 minutes. Garnish with remaining basil.

Recipe created by Mitzi. Reprinted with permission from Wal-Mart Stores, Inc. © 2013 Wal-Mart Stores, Inc.

Spice Rubbed Pork Tenderloin

Makes 6 servings

1 tablespoon cumin
1 tablespoon chili powder
2 teaspoons cinnamon
1 teaspoon red pepper flakes
1 teaspoon ground black pepper
2 pounds pork tenderloin

Preheat grill to a medium-high heat. Combine spices into 1-gallon resealable plastic bag. Seal and shake well to blend. Place tenderloins in bag and shake to evenly distribute the rub. Place pork on the grill for 15 to 20 minutes. You'll want a final temperature of 160°F, leaving the center pink and juicy. You can cook until 145°F and allow to set for an additional 10 minutes before slicing; the temperature of the tenderloin will continue to rise while the juices redistribute throughout the meat.

Taco Pizza

Makes 6 servings

1 lb. lean ground beef
½ package low-sodium taco seasoning
1 12-inch round whole wheat pizza dough
1 can (16 oz.) nonfat refried beans
2 medium tomatoes, chopped
½ cup part-skim mozzarella cheese
½ cup cheddar cheese
Extras:
Light sour cream
Salsa

Preheat oven to 350°F. In a nonstick skillet, brown beef over medium heat with taco seasoning according to package directions. Spray a pizza pan with nonstick cooking spray. Place whole wheat pizza dough on pizza pan. Cover with a layer of non-fat refried beans. Put beef on pizza and then sprinkle with both cheeses. Bake for about 12-15 minutes or until cheese melts. Top with tomatoes. Serve with salsa and light sour cream if desired.

Whole Wheat Tortellini and Shrimp Salad

Makes 6 servings

1 package (9 oz.) Buitoni refrigerated whole wheat Three Cheese Tortellini
20 large shrimp, cooked
½ cup halved grape or cherry tomatoes
¼ cup low-fat Greek dressing
3 tablespoons crumbled feta cheese

Prepare pasta according to package directions, then put in large bowl and refrigerate 10 minutes. Add cooked shrimp, tomatoes, dressing, and cheese. Toss and serve.

Sides

Balsamic Baby Carrots

Makes 4 servings

1 lb. Grimmway Farms baby carrots
2 teaspoon olive oil
1/4 cup balsamic vinegar

Preheat oven to 400°F. In an 8 x 8 baking dish, toss carrots with olive oil. Roast by occasionally stirring until tender, about 20 minutes. Drizzle balsamic vinegar and shake pan to coat evenly. Roast another 5 to 10 minutes, until carrots are tender golden and glazed.

Kale Chips

These make a delicious snack, too!
Makes 3 servings

5 oz. kale, cut and rinsed
1 tablespoon olive oil
Sea salt, to taste

Preheat oven to 350°F. On a 9 x 13 nonstick sheet cake pan spread the kale evenly in a single layer. Sprinkle the olive oil and sea salt on top. Bake 12 minutes or to your desired crispiness.

Lemon Parmesan Kale Salad

Makes 2 servings

1 bunch of kale, chopped
1 teaspoon extra virgin olive oil
juice from one lemon
3 tablespoons of shaved Parmesan cheese

Rinse kale thoroughly. Place in stockpot with about 2 tablespoons water on low heat for 12 to 15 minutes, until kale wilts. Add olive oil and toss to coat. Sprinkle with lemon juice and top with Parmesan cheese.

Microwave-Baked Sweet Potato

Makes 1 serving

1 sweet potato
dash of cinnamon
1 teaspoon honey

Wash sweet potato well, but leave the skin on. Using a fork, poke several holes through the skin. Place the sweet potato on a paper towel in the microwave and place another paper towel loosely over its top. Cook on high for 6 to 8 minutes. To test doneness, give the sweet potato a gentle squeeze. If it "gives" a little, then it's done. If not, cook another 1 to 2 minutes and test again. Cool for 3 to 4 minutes. Sprinkle with cinnamon and drizzle with honey.

Parmesan Roasted Asparagus

Makes 4 servings

1 bunch of asparagus
1 teaspoon olive oil
3 tablespoons Parmesan cheese
Sea salt, to taste
juice from one lemon

Preheat oven to 400°F. Spray a baking sheet with nonstick cooking spray. Place the asparagus, olive oil, and Parmesan inside a gallon-size resealable plastic bag and shake to coat asparagus. Spread asparagus on the baking sheet in a single layer. Roast until tender, about 10 to 12 minutes. Sprinkle with lemon juice and serve.

Pistachio Cranberry Freekeh Salad

Makes 8 servings

1 cup freekeh
½ cup pistachios
½ cup dried cranberries
2 tablespoons balsamic vinegar
½ cup feta cheese

Combine 2½ cups of water with freekeh in a saucepan and bring to a boil. Cover, reduce heat, and simmer 16 to 20 minutes. Gently stir in pistachios, cranberries, and balsamic vinegar. Top with feta cheese. Serve warm or cold.

Quinoa Fruit Salad

Makes 2 servings

½ cup quinoa
1 cup water
5 California strawberries, sliced
1 peach, cut into cubes
½ cup blueberries

Dressing:
1 tablespoon honey
1 tablespoon lemon juice

In a medium saucepan over medium heat, bring the quinoa and water to boil. Once it boils, reduce to simmer and cook with the lid on for about 12 to 14 minutes, until most of the water has been absorbed. Remove from heat, fluff with a fork, and cool. In a small bowl, mix together honey and lemon juice. Set aside. Mix together cooled quinoa with fruit and top with dressing.

Skinny Strawberry Salad

Makes 4 serving

1 pound mixed romaine
1 pint California strawberries
4 ounces crumbled bleu cheese
1/2 cup pecans, chopped (optional)

Dressing:
3 tablespoons extra virgin olive oil
2 tablespoons sugar
½ cup red wine vinegar
1 clove garlic, minced

Cut the greens, slice the strawberries, and place in refrigerator. Toast the pecans at 350°F for about 5 minutes, then set aside. Mix dressing ingredients together and set aside. When ready to serve, mix all ingredients together.

Steamed Spinach

Makes 4 Servings

1 pound baby spinach leaves, washed well and drained
Sea salt to taste
½ lemon, juiced

Put spinach in stockpot and sprinkle with 1 tablespoon water. Cook over medium heat for 5 to 6 minutes, allowing the spinach to cook down. Then sprinkle lightly with sea salt and lemon juice.

Sweet Potato Casserole

Makes 8 servings

3 cups mashed cooked sweet potatoes (about 2 pounds)
⅓ cup 1% organic milk
2 egg whites, lightly beaten
1 teaspoon vanilla
¾ cup brown sugar
¼ cup whole wheat flour
2 tablespoons butter
¼ cup pecans

Preheat oven to 350°F. Casserole: Combine the sweet potatoes, milk, egg whites, vanilla, and ¼ cup of the brown sugar in a bowl. Spray an 8-inch square baking dish with nonstick cooking spray and pour the mixture into the dish.
Topping: Combine the remaining ½ cup of brown sugar with the whole wheat flour. Use a pastry blender or a fork to mix in the butter. Once the mixture is crumbly, stir in the pecans. Sprinkle the topping mixture onto the casserole and bake for 30 minutes.

Watermelon Feta Salad

Makes 1 serving

1 cup watermelon, cut into cubes
1 tablespoon feta cheese
2 teaspoons chopped fresh basil or mint

Mix watermelon, feta, and basil in a bowl. Serve chilled.

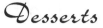Desserts

Lots of these tasty treats can do double duty in your kitchen: They make delicious snacks, too!

Frozen Banana Peanut Butter Bites

Makes 3 servings

3 medium ripe bananas
¼ cup Great Value natural creamy peanut butter

Peel one banana. Mash half of the peeled banana with the peanut butter. Set aside the mixture. Peel the other 2 bananas. Cut the unused ½ banana and other 2 bananas lengthwise into ½-inch slices. Put the mixture on half and then place the other banana half on top, making banana sandwiches. Freeze for 2 hours.

Frozen Greek Yogurt Banana Pops

Makes 6 servings

3 ripe bananas
¾ cup Great Value Greek Nonfat Vanilla Yogurt
6 tablespoons sliced almonds
6 Popsicle sticks

Cut bananas in half. Insert sticks into bananas. Roll bananas into Greek yogurt. Cover each banana with sliced almonds. Freeze for at least 2 hours.

Greek Yogurt Covered California Strawberries

Makes 3 servings

6 California strawberries
½ cup nonfat Greek vanilla yogurt

Place a piece of wax paper on a countertop. Put the Greek yogurt in a wide bowl. Dip the strawberries into the yogurt, twisting each one in a circle to create a smooth, evenly distributed coat of Greek yogurt. Place them on the wax paper and put in freezer for at least 2 hours.

Recipe created by Mitzi. Reprinted with permission from California Strawberry Commission.

Peach Crumble

Makes 9 servings

6 ripe peaches, peeled, pitted, and sliced
¼ cup whole wheat flour
¼ cup brown sugar
¼ cup quick cooking oats
juice of a lemon
2 tablespoons butter, room temperature

Greek Yogurt Mixture
½ cup non-fat Greek yogurt
1 tablespoon brown sugar

Preheat oven to 375°F. Combine Greek yogurt and 1 tablespoon brown sugar in a bowl; stir well. Cover and refrigerate at least 30 minutes. Spray an 8-inch square baking dish with nonstick cooking spray. Place sliced peaches in pan and sprinkle with lemon juice. Combine flour, sugar, oats, lemon juice, and butter. Mix together until crumbly. Sprinkle crumb mixture evenly over peaches. Bake 30 minutes or until peaches are soft and topping is lightly browned. Top with Greek yogurt mixture.

Peanut Butter Honey Greek Yogurt Dip

Makes 3 servings

1 (6 oz.) container of plain Greek yogurt
1 tablespoon honey
1 tablespoon peanut butter
½ teaspoon cinnamon
Assorted fruits such as strawberries, bananas, or apples for dipping

Mix the first four ingredients until well blended. Serve with fruit dippers.

Skinny "Fried" Honey Bananas

Makes 2 servings

1 banana
1 tablespoon honey
¼ teaspoon cinnamon

Slice banana to about ⅛ inch thick. In a small bowl, mix honey together with 2 teaspoons of water; set aside. Heat a nonstick skillet to medium heat and spray with nonstick cooking spray. Add banana slices to skillet. Once browned (about 4 to 5 minutes), flip to other side. Let bananas cook for 1 to 2 minutes more, then turn off stove and drizzle the honey and water mixture on top. Mixture will bubble. Turn bananas over to brown both sides. Sprinkle with cinnamon.

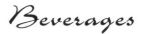

Beverages

Skinny Strawberry Sangria

Makes 10 servings

1 bottle (750 ml) red wine
2 cans (12 oz.) lime-flavored LaCroix Sparkling Water,
3 cups California strawberries, hulled and sliced lengthwise

Add 2 cups of the sliced strawberries to a large pitcher. Pour the wine over the strawberries. Cover, place in refrigerator for 4 to 5 hours. Remove from refrigerator and add lime sparkling water and a few handfuls of ice. Add the remaining strawberries to glasses. Pour the sangria over the strawberries.

> Recipe created by Mitzi. Reprinted with permission from California Strawberry Commission.

Cherry Berry Punch

Makes 1 serving
This is one of my favorite holiday drinks.

6 oz. cran-raspberry-flavored LaCroix Sparkling Water
1 to 2 oz. tart cherry juice
frozen berries

Fill half your glass with chilled cran-raspberry-flavored sparkling water. Top with tart cherry juice. Stir gently. Add berries to garnish.

Skinny Prosecco

Makes 1 serving

4 oz. pure LaCroix sparkling water
2 oz. Prosecco wine
2 California strawberries, sliced in half

Fill a champagne flute with chilled sparkling water. Top with Prosecco. Add two strawberries to garnish.

Strawberry Watermelon Lemonade

Makes 1 serving

½ cup watermelon
3 California strawberries
4 oz. lemon-flavored LaCroix sparkling water
1 oz. lemon juice
1 lemon wedge

Blend together watermelon and strawberries. Pour into glass and top with lemon sparkling water and lemon juice. Stir gently. For a garnish, add a lemon wedge to the rim of the glass.

Skinny Cape Cod

Makes 1 serving

6 oz. lime-flavored LaCroix sparkling water
1 oz. vodka
1 oz. cranberry juice

Fill glass with lime-flavored sparkling water. Add vodka and cranberry juice. Stir gently.

Spice It Up

Spices can make ordinary dishes extraordinary with a simple pinch, dash, or shake. But they do much more than add vibrant color and kick to our food. Spices are packed with natural antioxidants—the same stuff that makes fruits and vegetables so good for you. Antioxidants boost your immune system and your metabolism, curb your appetite, and reduce inflammation, which helps to prevent heart disease, cancer, diabetes, and other chronic diseases.

Here are a few of my faves:

Cinnamon: Keep a shaker of ground cinnamon handy to sprinkle over everything from hot cocoa to smoothies, oatmeal, and fruit salad.

Ginger: Sweeten 1 cup of hot or iced tea with ¼ teaspoon of Ground Ginger mixed with 1 teaspoon honey

Thyme and oregano: Wake up your taste buds with herbed scrambled eggs: Beat ⅛ teaspoon of thyme or oregano leaves into 2 eggs before scrambling.

CHAPTER 11:

THE PINTEREST DIET WORKOUT: A 30-DAY EXERCISE PLAN

"Difficult doesn't mean impossible.
It simply means that you have to work hard."
—Anonymous

F ollowing *The Pinterest Diet* Workout program, you'll get results you've never seen before. Best of all, it doesn't take a lot of time to deliver those amazing results! That's because I've designed the workout for maximum efficiency. In other words, you'll be working out for shorter amounts of time, but at a high-intensity level that lets you burn more calories and exercise more effectively.

> Reminder! Before beginning any exercise program, get your doctor's approval. Make sure he or she has no objection to you participating in a high-intensity interval-training program. *The Pinterest Diet* Workout program is designed for people who don't have any medical conditions or physical limitations.

HIIT And Tabata Training Method

How does it work? *The Pinterest Diet* Workout Program is a complete high-intensity interval-training (HIIT) program that includes my favorite calorie-torching, fat-burning methods as well as what I consider a fitness miracle: Tabata Interval Training. Again, think highly effective and efficient workouts.

Founded in Japan in the 1970s by Dr. Izumi Tabata for the country's Olympians, Tabata training involves doing a series of eight ultra-high-intensity exercises for 20 seconds with 10-second rests between them—for a total of four minutes. The moves are simple, but the pace is challenging.

Praised by both scientific researchers and fitness experts, Tabata training is an extremely efficient way to boost your aerobic and anaerobic capacity and improve your resting metabolic rate. It also allows you to burn more fat in less time. Studies show that 27 minutes of high-intensity interval training (HIIT) three times per week produces the same anaerobic and aerobic improvement as 60 minutes of cardio five times per week.

I owned and operated a boot camp, and I started including Tabata training for my boot campers about four years ago. They loved the simplicity of it and the incredible results they saw. So will you!

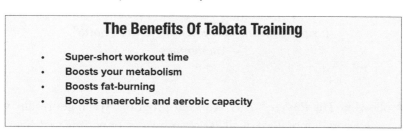

The Benefits Of Tabata Training

- **Super-short workout time**
- **Boosts your metabolism**
- **Boosts fat-burning**
- **Boosts anaerobic and aerobic capacity**

"A one-hour workout is 4% of your day. No excuses."
—Anonymous

The Exercise Program
The Basics:

- Work out at least three times a week for 12 to 30 minutes each time.
- Visit my Workout Plans Board for additional ideas and photos of different exercises and stretches.
- Always push yourself to work out at your own maximum-intensity level.
- If you're unsure how to do any of the exercises in *The Pinterest Diet* Workout, just check the Exercise Glossary at the end of the chapter. I've included easy step-by-step instructions for all of them.

How To Do A Tabata

- Do the exercise for 20 seconds, pushing yourself to your maximum intensity level.
- Rest for 10 seconds.
- Repeat the sequence 7 times.

In total, you'll be doing 8 workout/rest intervals, for a total time of 4 minutes. When you start Tabata training, you might not be able to complete all 8 intervals or the full 20 seconds. Don't worry. Just work to the best of your ability and do as much as you can. You'll improve every time you work out. Increase your intensity level as your fitness level improves. You'll be amazed at how quickly you'll gain strength and stamina while shedding body fat.

The Five-Minute Warm-up
Do this five-minute warm-up before every workout.

- 1 minute High Knees in place
- 1 minute Butt Kicks in place
- 1 minute Jumping Jacks
- 1 minute Jogging in place
- 1 minute Seal Jacks

How To Read The Exercise Program

Read all exercises from left to right, for example, start with 10 sprints, then 20 walking lunges, then 30 seconds rest. Where you see (1 x 10) following an exercise, it means you should do one set of 10.

Week 1: Day 1

10 Sprints	20 Walking Lunges
30 seconds rest	20 Walking Lunges
Double Arm Rows (1 x 10)	Shoulder Presses (1 x 10)
Bent-over Lateral Raises (1 x 10)	30 seconds rest
Double Arm Rows (1 x 10)	Shoulder Presses (1 x 10)
Bent-over Lateral Raises (1 x 10)	Star Jump Tabata (8 intervals of 20 seconds each with 10-second breaks between)
Bicep Curls (1 x 10)	Hammer Curls (1 x 10)
In/out Bicep Curls (1 x 10)	30 seconds rest
Bicep Curls (1 x 10)	Hammer Curls (1 x 10)
In/out Bicep Curls (1 x 10)	Jump Squat Tabata
45-second Standing Plank Hold	150 Crunches

> Sprints can be done in your yard, a parking lot, a track, a treadmill—or just by jogging fast in place for 10 seconds and counting it as one sprint. If you're going from one spot to another, your sprint should be about 100 feet or 33 yards.

Day 2

25 Jumping Jacks	5 Push-ups
8 Burpees	25 Crunches
25 High Knees	5 Push-ups
10 Jump Squats	25 Crunches
60 second Wall Sit	10 Star Jumps
25 High Knees	25 Jumping Jacks
Repeat all exercises 2 more times.	

Day 3

20 Walking Lunges	30 seconds rest
20 Walking Lunges	30 seconds rest
20 Walking Lunges-30 seconds rest	Mountain Climber Tabata
12 Sprints	Tricep Push-ups (1 x 10)
Skullcrushers (1 x 10)	Tricep Kickbacks (1 x 10)
Tricep Dips (1 x 10)	30 seconds rest
Tricep Push-ups (1 x 10)	Skullcrushers (1 x 10)
Tricep Kickbacks (1 x 10)	Tricep Dips (1 x 10)
30 seconds rest	Tricep Push-ups (1 x 10)
Skullcrushers (1 x 10)	Tricep Kickbacks (1 x 10)
Tricep Dips (1 x 10)	30 seconds rest
Burpee Tabata	200 Crunches of your choice

Week 2: Day 1

20 Walking Lunges with 5-lb. weights in each hand at 90 degrees
30 seconds rest
20 Walking Lunges with 5-lb. weights in each hand at 90 degrees
30 seconds rest
20 Walking Lunges with 5-lb. weights in each hand at 90 degrees
30 seconds rest

Pendulum Tabata	Push-ups (1 x 10)
Tricep Push-ups (1 x 10)	Wide Push-ups (1 x 10)
Star Jump Tabata	Push-ups (1 x 10)
Tricep Push-ups (1 x 10)	Wide Push-ups (1 x 10)
Mountain Climber Tabata	Push-ups (1 x 10)
Tricep Push-ups (1 x 10)	Wide Push-ups (1 x 10)
60 seconds rest	(1 x 10)(1 x 10)
Dumbbell Thruster Tabata	Push-ups (1 x 10)
Tricep Push-ups (1 x 10)	Wide Push-ups (1 x 10)

Day 2

20 Walking Lunges with 5-lb. weights in each hand at 90 degrees	
30 seconds rest	
20 Walking Lunges with 5-lb. weights in each hand at 90 degrees	
30 seconds rest	
20 Walking Lunges with 5-lb. weights in each hand at 90 degrees	
30 seconds rest	
Jump Squat Tabata	Overhead Tricep Extensions (1 x 10)
Hammer Curls (1 x 10)	In/out Bicep Curls (1 x 10)
(1 x 10)-30 seconds rest	Overhead Tricep Extensions (1 x 10)
Hammer Curls (1 x 10)	In/out Bicep Curls (1 x 10)
Burpee Tabata	Double-armed Rows (1 x 10)
Bent-over Lateral Raises (1 x 10)	Front Raises (1 x 10)
30 seconds rest	Double-armed Row (1 x 10)
Bent-over Lateral Raises (1 x 10)	Front Raises (1 x 10)
Star Jumps (1 x 10)	Jump-ups (1 x 10)
Standing Plank (90 seconds)	100 Jumping Jacks
300 Crunches	

Day 3

Sprints (15)	1-minute exercises:
(Do each of the following for 60 seconds.)	
Switch Kicks	Full Body Crunches
Jump Squats	Pec Decs
Shoulder Shrugs	Mountain Climber Push-ups (2 Mountain Climbers/2 Push-ups)

Hammer Curls	60 seconds rest
Tricep Push-ups	Pendulums
Alternating split-squat Jumps	Bent-over Lateral Raises
Mountain Climbers	Prisoner Squats
Star Jump Burpees	Tricep Kickbacks
Squat Hops	Calf Raises
Bicep Curls	Reverse Crunches
Standing Squats, Tabata style	Wide Push-ups
Monkey Push-ups	

Week 3: Day 1

20 Walking Lunges with 5- to 8-lb. weights in each hand at 90 degrees	
30 seconds rest	
20 Walking Lunges with 5- to 8-lb. weights in each hand at 90 degrees	
30 seconds rest	
20 Walking Lunges with 5- to 8-lb. weights in each hand at 90 degrees	
30 seconds rest	
Tricep Dips (1 x 10)	Tricep Push-ups (1 x 10)
Skullcrushers (1 x 10)	Push-up Blaster Tabata
30 seconds rest	Tricep Dips (1 x 10)
Tricep Push-ups (1 x 10)	Skullcrushers (1 x 10)
Burpee Tabata	Bicycles (90 seconds)
250 Crunches	

Day 2

Jump Squat Tabata	Bicep In/out 1 x 10
Hammer Curls (1 x 10)	Crossover Curls (1 x 10)
Mountain Climber Tabata	Bicep In/out (1 x 10)
Hammer Curls (1 x 10)	Crossover Curls (1 x 10)
Star Jump Tabata	Bicep In/out (1 x 10)
Hammer Curls (1 x 10)	Crossover Curls (1 x 10)
Burpee Tabata	Push-ups (1 x 10)
Wide Push-ups (1 x 10)	

Day 3

20 Walking Lunges with 5- to 8-lb. weights in each hand at 90 degrees	
30 seconds rest	
20 Walking Lunges with 5- to 8-lb. weights in each hand at 90 degrees	
30 seconds rest	
20 Walking Lunges with 5- to 8-lb. weights in each hand at 90 degrees	
30 seconds rest	
Sprints (20)	Star Jump Burpee Tabata
Prisoner Squats (1 x 10)	Tricep Kickbacks (1 x 10)
Jump Squats (1 x 10)	Pec Decs (1 x 10)
Shoulder Shrugs (1 x 10)	Mountain Climber Push-ups (2 Mountain Climbers/2 Push-ups) Tabata
Hammer Curls (1 x 10)	Tricep Push-ups (1 x 10)
Pendulums (1 x 10)	Alternating Split Squat Jumps (1 x 10)
Bent-over Lateral Raises (1 x 10)	

Week 4: Day 1

20 Walking Lunges with 5- to 8-lb. weights in each hand at 90 degrees	
30 seconds rest	
20 Walking Lunges with 5- to 8-lb. weights in each hand at 90 degrees	
30 seconds rest	
20 Walking Lunges with 5- to 8-lb. weights in each hand at 90 degrees	
30 seconds rest	
Dumbbell Thruster Tabata	30 seconds rest
Tricep Push-ups (1 x 10)	Skullcrushers (1 x 10)
Burpee Tabata	30 seconds rest
Tricep Push-ups (1 x 10)	Skullcrushers (1 x 10)
Tabata Style Squat Tabata	Full Standing Plank (90 seconds)
25 Full-body Crunches	

Day 2

Push-up Blaster Tabata	Pec Decs (1 x 10)
Regular Push-ups (1 x 10)	Jump Squat Tabata
Double-armed Rows (1 x 10)	Front Raises (1 x 10)

Bent-over Lateral Raises (1 x 10)	Push-up Blaster Tabata
Pec Decs (1 x 10)	Regular Push-ups (1 x 10)
Burpee with Star Jump Tabata	Double-armed Rows (1 x 10)
Front Raises (1 x 10)	Bent-over Lateral Raises (1 x 10)
100 Bicycles (100 to each side)	

Day 3

20 Walking Lunges with 5- to 8-lb. weights in each hand at 90 degrees	
30 seconds rest	
20 Walking Lunges with 5- to 8-lb. weights in each hand at 90 degrees	
30 seconds rest	
20 Walking Lunges with 5- to 8-lb. weights in each hand at 90 degrees	
30 seconds rest	
25 Jump Squats	25 Star Jumps
25 Jumping Jacks	25 Air Jumps
45 seconds rest	25 Burpees
25 Seal Jacks	25 Squat Hops
25 Dumbbell Thrusters	25 Standing Pendulums (25 each side)
45 seconds rest	25 Star Jumps
25 Jumping Jacks	25 Air Jumps
45 seconds rest	25 Burpees
25 Standing Pendulums (25 each side)	Standing Plank (90 seconds)
Full-body Crunches (60 seconds)	

Movement Munchies! A recent study in the *European Heart Journal* found that people who spend a lot of time sitting during the day have higher risks of obesity, metabolic syndrome, and heart disease. These risks are still there even for people who exercise. Whether you sit behind a desk, in front of a TV, or behind the wheel, I want you to aim to move for five minutes every hour to help you stay slim and healthy. The study suggested getting up and moving around often and taking breaks as short as one minute can improve your health.

Take a break and slim your waist! Check out my Movement Munchies Board on Pinterest to get ideas for what you can do for five minutes every hour. Even if you exercise regularly, you'll still benefit by adding these mini workouts to your routine.

Optional Additional Workouts

If you want to work out more than three times a week, try the following routines. They're a fun way to add variety to your exercise regimen. Plus, they're super-short, so if you're pressed for time, they're a great option.

12-Minute Workout Option 1
> Star Jump Tabata
> Jump Squat Tabata
> Switch Kick Tabata

12-Minute Workout Option 2
> Side Plank Jump Tabata
> Switch Kick Tabata
> Mountain Climber Tabata

12-Minute Workout Option 3
> Squat Hop Tabata
> Dumbbell Thruster Tabata
> Burpee with Star Jump Tabata

Mitzi's Super-Short Sizzle
> This workout is intended for times when you have literally five minutes. You can do it in your own home. And, it only takes four minutes, so you'll have a minute to spare!
>
> Tabata of your choice (jump squat, star jump, burpee, dumbbell thruster, mountain climbers, etc.)

Need Something Tougher?

If you're ready for a serious physical and mental challenge, try my 1000 Challenge workout with 100 of the following 10 exercises. But, be warned: I call it a "challenge" for a reason.

1000 Challenge Workout

100 jump Squats	100 Reach-ups
100 Mountain Climbers	100 Tricep Dips
100 Air Jumps	100 Walking Lunges
100 Burpees	100 Bicycles
100 Star Jumps	100 Squats

Muffin-Top Workout

50 Crunches	20 V-ups
50 Reverse Crunches	1 minute Standing Plank
15 Full-body Crunches	20 Oblique Crunches (left side)
20 Oblique Crunches (right side)	Repeat 2 to 3 times.

Breathing Tip:

Here's an easy way to remember proper breathing while weight training: Always exhale when you exert the force.

"I hated every minute of training, but I said, "Don't quit. Suffer now and live the rest of your life as a champion"
—Muhammad Ali

Exercise Glossary

Need a visual? I've got diagrams, photos, and videos of lots of these exercises on my Pinterest boards. So, if you need more guidance, just log on!

> **TIP:** When you first start the exercise program, you will be doing the 7-Day Jumpstart Cleanse so your calorie intake will be reduced. The ideal time to workout would be about 1-2 hours after you have eaten one of your meals to help boost your energy levels. If you need an exercise boost prior to your workout and can't eat a meal, you can make a "mini" one of my smoothie recipes. This means you simply divide all the ingredients in half.

Air Jumps: Act like you're jumping rope without really jumping a rope. Rotate hands quickly and take small quick jumps.

Alternating Split Squat Jumps: Start in a split stance with one leg in front of the other. Squat down, then jump up as high as possible and switch back leg to front position, and front leg to back as quickly as possible in midair. Begin next jump immediately upon landing. Make sure your knee does not go beyond 90 degree angle. Your knee should be above your ankle.

Bent-over Lateral Raises: Holding dumbbells in each hand, stand with your feet hip-width apart and slightly bend your knees. Fold your torso forward, keeping your back straight and almost parallel to the floor. Dangle your arms down toward the floor and lift them to the sides so they are in line with your shoulders, keeping a slight bend in the elbows. Then slowly lower the dumbbells back to the starting position.

Bicep Curls: Standing with feet hip-width apart, hold dumbbells in each hand and face palms outwards in front of you. Slowly contract your arms up toward your chest. Slowly lower them back to the starting position.

Bicycles: Lie face-up with your hips and knees bent 90 degrees so your lower legs are parallel to the floor. Place your hands behind your head. Lift your shoulders off the floor and hold them there. Twist your upper body to the left as you pull your left knee in as fast as you can until it touches your left elbow. Simultaneously straighten your right leg. Return to the starting position and repeat to the other side.

Burpees: Stand with your feet shoulder width apart and your arms at your sides. Push your hips back, bend your knees, and lower your body into as deep a squat as possible. Then, kick your legs backward, so that you are in a push-up position. Do a push-up, then quickly bring your legs back to the squat position. Stand up quickly and jump. Repeat.

Burpee with Star Jumps: Stand with your feet shoulder-width apart and your arms at your sides. Push your hips back, bend your knees, and lower your body into as deep a squat as possible. Then, kick legs backward, so that you are in a push-up position. Do a push-up, then quickly bring your legs back to the squat position. Stand up quickly and do a star jump. Repeat.

Calf Raises: Stand up straight, with your feet hip-width apart. Slowly raise your heels until you're on your tiptoes and balance your weight on the balls of your feet. Pause briefly and then slowly lower yourself. Repeat.

> Interval timers are an easy way to time your workouts for Tabatas. You can buy one at GymBoss.com or download a free interval timer on your smartphone.

Chest Flies: Holding two dumbbells, lie face-up on the floor or a bench. Hold your arms straight above your chest, with your arms slightly bent. Rotate your shoulders until your elbows point outwards. Lower the dumbbells to your sides until your arms are parallel to the ground. Bring the dumbbells back together above your chest.

Concentrated Bicep Curls: Sit or kneel and hold a dumbbell in your right hand. Bend forward, keeping your abs engaged and prop your right elbow against the inside of your right thigh. Contract your bicep and curl your hand toward your shoulder without moving your elbow. Lower your right arm all the way down to starting position. Repeat, using the left arm.

Crossover Curls: Start in a standing position with a dumbbell in each hand. Press the dumbbells high above your head, palms facing each other. Keeping your elbows stationary, lower your left forearm behind your head, near your right ear. Press the dumbbell back into the starting position and repeat with your right arm.

Crunches: Lie on your back with your knees bent and your feet flat on the floor. Place your hands behind your ears. Keep your lower back on the floor and curl your shoulders forward by slowly lifting your shoulders, head, and upper back. While doing this, tense your abdominal muscles and hold for 3 to 4 seconds. Slowly return to the starting position.

Double Arm Rows: Stand with your feet together with dumbbells in your hands. Bend your knees and hinge forward from your hips. Your back should be flat. Your arms will hang in a straight line toward the ground. Pull the dumbbells toward your abdomen, squeezing your shoulder blades together. Then slowly release the weights and return to the starting position.

Dumbbell Thrusters: Hold a pair of dumbbells with your arms bent in front of your shoulders with your palms facing each other. Position your feet shoulder-width apart, then quickly lower your hips until your thighs are parallel to the floor. Explode back up and push the dumbbells above your head until your arms are straight. Hold for one second, then lower the dumbbells and squat back down.

> **Weights:** For resistance training, pick a weight that you can lift comfortably for 10 to 12 reps. You should be struggling by the last few reps, but still be able to maintain good form.

Front Raises: Grasp a dumbbell in each hand. Position the dumbbells in front of your upper legs with your elbows slightly bent. Raise the dumbbells forward and upward with until your upper arms are horizontal. Lower your arms to the starting position.

Hammer Curls: Hold the dumbbells at your sides, with your palms facing and your arms straight. With your elbows to your sides, raise one dumbbell until your forearm is vertical and your thumb faces your shoulder. Lower it to the starting position and repeat with the other arm.

In/out Bicep Curls: Stand with feet shoulder-width apart. Bend your knees slightly and position your arms down by your sides with your shoulders back. With a dumbbell in each hand and your palms facing forward, bend your elbows and bring each dumbbell up to your shoulders. Return to the starting position. Before your next repetition, rotate your arms at the shoulders so that your palms rotate farther away from your body. You're your elbows and bring the dumbbells back up to your shoulders. Then slowly return to the starting position. Alternate between these two positions.

Jumping Jacks: Stand with your feet together and your hands at your sides. Simultaneously extend your arms above your head and jump up while spreading your feet out wide. Quickly reverse the movement. Bounce on the balls of your feet.

Modified Push-ups: Position yourself as if you were going to do a regular push-up, but put your knees on the ground about hip-distance apart. Keep your back straight and movement controlled as you raise and lower your torso.

Monkey Push-ups: Start out standing and slowly lower your torso forward until your hands hit the floor. Your knees will be slightly bent and your rear will be in the air. Lower yourself to do a push-up and then immediately jump straight up, keeping your arms down at your sides. Repeat.

> Foam rollers are an excellent way to reduce stress and get a good stretch any time. It's also a perfect Movement Munchie. I keep one in my office and one in my bedroom. Go to my Movement Munchies Board and check out the How to Foam Roll Like a Pro repin: pinterest.com/pin/186266134561305623/.

Overhead Tricep Extensions: While sitting, place a dumbbell above your head with both hands under the inner plate. With your elbows over your head, lower your forearms by bending your elbows. Keep your wrists flexed to prevent letting the dumbbell hit your neck. Raise the dumbbell above your head by extending your elbows and return to the starting position.

Full-body Crunches: Lay on your back on the floor or a mat. Raise your knees in the air so that your thighs are perpendicular to your upper body and the ground. Bend your knees, raise your head off the ground slightly, and place both your hands behind your head. Raise your upper body toward your legs and raise your legs toward your chest at the same time.

Jump Squats: Stand with your arms at your sides and your knees bent slightly. Dip your knees and squat down to get ready to jump. Then, jump explosively as high as you can. When you land, immediately squat down and jump again.

Mountain Climbers: Place your hands on the floor a little wider than shoulder-width. Stand on the balls of your feet, position one leg forward, bent under your body, and extend the other leg back. Keeping your upper body in place, alternate leg positions by pushing your hips up while extending your forward leg backward and pulling rear leg forward under your body. Land on both feet simultaneously.

Oblique Crunches: Lie on your back with your knees bent and your feet flat on the floor. Slowly drop your legs to the left and let your knees rest near the floor. Place your hands behind your ears. Push your lower back into the floor, flattening the arch and hold. Slowly curl up so that both your shoulders lift off the floor a few inches. Hold briefly and lower to the starting position. Repeat and then switch to the other side.

Pec Decs: Standing with your feet about shoulder-width apart, hold a dumbbell in each hand. Start out with your arms bent to a 90-degree angle at the elbows, your palms facing forward, and your hands directly above your elbows. Slowly move your elbows together but never let them touch. Keep your hands directly above your elbows at all times. Slowly move back to the starting position and repeat.

Pendulums: Put your hands on the ground and swing your right leg out to the side. Use your left toe and your hands to support your body. Bring your right leg back to the starting position. Repeat the movement with your left leg. Continue to alternate legs.

Prisoner Squats: Stand with your feet slightly more than shoulder-width apart. Keep your back straight and your chest out. Lace your fingers behind your head, with your elbows out. Slowly lower your body until you are in a squat position with your thighs parallel to the floor. Make sure your knees do not extend beyond your toes. Pause and then push back up into the starting position.

Push-ups: Assume a plank position, so that your hands and toes are supporting your weight, with your hands slightly wider than your shoulders. Keeping your upper and lower body straight and moving as one unit, use your arms to lower your body until your chest nearly touches the floor. Push yourself back up as quickly as possible.

Push-up Blasters: Start with your hands and feet on the ground and your knees bent. Jump back into a standing plank position (see definition) with your feet about hip-distance apart. Then, quickly and simultaneously move both your legs to a wide position, do a push-up, then bring your legs back to hip-distance apart. Return to the starting position, with your feet almost under your hips. Repeat.

Reach-ups: Lie on your back with your legs straight up. Cross your left ankle over your right. Keep your shoulders on the ground and your whole lower body still. Tighten your abs. Reach both hands up while holding one dumbbell. Slowly lower and raise the dumbbell while maintaining contracted abs.

Reverse Crunches: Lie on the floor and place your hands on the floor or behind your head. Bring your knees in toward your chest until they are bent at a 90-degree angle to your body, with your feet together or crossed. Contract your abs to curl your hips off the floor, reaching your legs up toward the ceiling. Lower your legs and repeat. Avoid swinging your legs for momentum.

Seal Jacks: Stand with your feet together and your arms extended in front of you at chest height. Simultaneously spread your arms out to the sides as you jump just enough to spread your feet wide. Without pausing, quickly reverse the movement. Keep your ankles locked and land on the balls of your feet.

Shoulder Presses: Hold a dumbbell in each hand. Position them so that they're level with your shoulders, with your elbows directly below your wrists. Press the dumbbells upward until your arms are fully extended. Slowly lower them back to the starting position.

Shoulder Shrugs: Stand holding dumbbells at your sides. Elevate your shoulders as high as possible and then return to the starting position.

Side Plank Jumps: Start in a standing plank position (see definition). Jump both feet up on the right side, then return to standing plank. Repeat the motion, jumping to the left side, then return to standing plank. When you jump to the sides, your knees will be bent.

Skaters: Cross your left leg behind your right leg as you bend your right knee 90 degrees. Extend your right arm out to your side and swing your left arm across your right leg. Jump a few feet to the left, repeating the motion in reverse. Repeat, simulating the movements of a speed skater.

Skullcrushers: Lie on the floor with a dumbbell in each hand. Position the dumbbell over your shoulders with your arms extended and perpendicular to the floor. Lower the dumbbells by bending your elbows and only moving your lower arms. Your upper arms are stationary throughout the exercise. Extend your arms, returning to the starting position.

Squat Hops: Stand with your feet shoulder-width apart. Lower yourself into a very low squat, with your back straight and your feet fully on the floor. Raise up onto your toes and hop 2 to 3 inches into the air while maintaining your squat position. Repeat this action.

Standing Pendulums: In a standing position, swing your right leg out to the side and back. Repeat the motion with your left leg. Keep alternating legs, always keeping one leg off the ground.

Standing Plank: Position yourself as if you were at the top of a push-up—with your hands and toes supporting your weight. Keep your hands flat on the floor, positioned slightly wider than your shoulders. Your arms should be straight and your legs should be extended so that your body is in a straight line from your shoulders to your ankles. Contract your abs as if you were about to be punched in the stomach. Hold this position for the desired length of time.

Star Jumps: Begin with your feet shoulder-width apart and your arms close to your body. Squat down halfway to the ground, then jump as high as you can. At the peak of the jump, fully extend your entire body, spreading your arms and legs out away from your body. As you land, bring your limbs back in.

Stationary Lunges: Begin by standing comfortably with your hands on your hips. Step forward with your right leg and slowly lower your left leg until your knee gets close to the ground. Your right knee should bend to 90 degrees. Push yourself back up to the starting position and switch legs. Make sure you keep your knee directly above your ankle; don't let it extend beyond your toes.

Switch Kicks: Standing up, kick your left leg out in front of you, and, as you are bringing it back down, switch and kick your right leg so that during the entire exercise only one foot is on the ground. As you are kicking your leg out, pull your elbows back by your side. . Continue to switch back and forth. Contract your abs while doing the exercise.

Tabata-style Squats: Stand with your feet shoulder-width apart. Lower your body, keeping your knees above your ankles (avoid allowing your knees to go in front of your toes), as far as you can by pushing your hips back and bending your knees. At the same time, swing your arms in an "X" movement as you lower and raise your body.

Start with your arms crossed when you're standing upright and, as you lower your arms, swing them out to your sides. Do this movement as quickly as possible.

Tricep Push-ups: These are similar to regular Push-ups, but your hands should be closer together. When you lower your body, keep your elbows in at your sides to maintain tension on the tricep muscle. Push off and return to the starting position.

Tricep Kickbacks: Hold a dumbbell in each hand and bend forward at the hips so that your upper arms (from elbow to shoulder) are parallel to the ground. Keeping the upper portion of your arms still, extend your lower arms until they're parallel to the ground. Slowly return to the starting position.

Tricep Dips: Stand facing away from a sturdy chair or bench. Place your hands shoulder-width apart on the chair or bench and position your feet approximately hip-width apart with your legs bent. Straighten your arms, keeping a slight bend at the elbows to protect your joints. Slowly bend your elbows and lower your upper body until your arms are at 90 degrees. Keep your back close to the bench. Then, slowly push upward, straightening your arms and return to the starting position.

Upright Row: Grasp your dumbbells and bring your hands up with palms facing your body and elbows going out to the side. Pull the dumbbells toward your neck with your elbows leading. Allow your wrists to flex as the bar rises. Lower your arms and return to the starting position.

V-ups: Lie face-up on the floor or a mat. Put your hands over your head, touching the floor with your palms facing upward and your legs extended. Keeping your arms and legs straight, simultaneously raise both of them, reaching your hands toward your feet. Slowly return to the starting position.

Walking Lunges: Begin by standing comfortably, with your hands on your hips. Step forward with your right leg and slowly lower your left leg until your knee gets close to the ground. Your right knee should bend to 90 degrees. Now, step forward with your left leg into a walking lunge and repeat, moving forward with each lunge.

Wide Push-ups: Assume a traditional push-up position, but place your hands about six inches wider than shoulder-width on each side. Bend your arms at the elbows until they reach 90 degrees. Press up until your arms are fully extended.

Success Story: Laura Peterson

I started working with Laura Peterson in November of 2010, when she signed up for my boot camp fitness classes in Kansas City. Laura had always been active, playing sports in high school and college, and she belonged to a gym. She'd even hired a costly personal trainer and run some races. But despite all that, she'd never reached the weight or gotten the body she dreamed of. After giving birth to her second child, she was beginning to wonder if her goals were even achievable.

She wanted to lose weight, get stronger, and have more energy. But she was tired of crowded gym classes and boring exercise machines that got her nowhere. Boot camp turned out to be the perfect fit for her.

Best of all, it gave her the missing piece of the fitness puzzle: nutrition. I encouraged her to start keeping a food journal, logging her daily intake honestly so that she could start holding herself accountable. For the first time, she realized that she, like so many of my clients, had calorie amnesia.

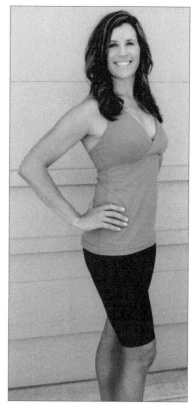

Mom of 3

She started adjusting her diet to get better nutrition and fewer empty calories. And, for the first time, she began to move away from the all-or-nothing diet attitude. "Mitzi helped me realize that I didn't have to be perfect when it came to dieting," Laura says. "I stopped beating myself up every time I enjoyed a couple of cocktails on the weekend or treated myself to an ice cream when I was buying one for my kids."

Laura took my boot camp class regularly, started doing Tabatas, and started eating clean. And she quickly reached her goal, shedding 15 excess pounds of fat, which was a loss of 9% body fat in seven months. She still exercises regularly and practices mindful eating.

"I feel happier with myself now, and my entire family eats healthier," says the mom of three, who will soon turn 40 but looks 30. "And I love the high-intensity interval training that Tabatas provide. I can work out for a shorter amount of time and still achieve great results!"

CHAPTER 12:

LIVING BETTER ON THE PINTEREST DIET

"A good laugh and a long sleep are the two best cures for anything."
—Irish proverb

Congratulations! You've made terrific progress in your journey toward better health in 30 days. You've made your 5 Transformation Boards and you're logging onto Pinterest every day. You've completed your 7-Day Jumpstart Cleanse. You've started *The Pinterest Diet* and *The Pinterest Diet* Workout. The goals you've always dreamed of reaching are closer than ever. Great job!

"People inspire you or they drain you. Pick them wisely."
—Hans F Hansen

There's one last missing piece you need to complete the puzzle. Let's call it the big-picture perspective. Healthy living is about more than just diet and exercise. It's about attitude, mindset, the way you approach every single day of your life. It's about what I call "mental nutrition." You have to nourish your mind just like you have to nourish your body. You can eat wholesome food and do Tabatas until your legs feel like jelly, but if you neglect other key components of the big picture, you'll still fall short. You won't be your best self.

In this chapter, we'll focus on three keys to better, happier, healthier living: laughter, sleep, and stress management. Each one of them plays a vital role in your quality of life and your ability to succeed on *The Pinterest Diet*—or in any other challenge you give yourself. Happily, there are some simple, proven strategies to improve all three areas of your life. Read on to find out how. And, as always, Pinterest can help. Be sure to check my boards regularly for the latest news on research breakthroughs, great new products, and more!

"Surround yourself with ONLY people
who are going to take you higher."
—*Oprah Winfrey*

Laughter: The Amazing Health Benefits Of LOL

Giggling. Chuckling. Splitting your sides. ROFL. Laughing is one of the fastest, most effective ways to bring your mind and body back into balance. But, unfortunately, most of us don't laugh nearly enough. Research shows that children laugh as much as 400 times every day. Adults, on the other hand, laugh only 15 to 17 times a day.

Why should you care? Because the old saying about laughter being the best medicine is TRUE. Laughing can improve your health in a multitude of ways.

Here are a few of the many health benefits of laughter.

Immunity Boost: When you laugh, your body produces more T cells, which boost your immunity to disease and make you less likely to catch colds and flus. One recent study found that watching funny videos increased people's production of beta-endorphins (chemicals that help block depression) and human growth hormone (which increases the body's immunity to disease) by as much as 87 percent.

Pain Relief: When you laugh, you release endorphins, the body's natural painkillers.

Mini Workout: Laughing not only relieves tension in your muscles, but when you laugh so hard your stomach and sides hurt, you exercise your diaphragm, which contracts your abdominals. It's almost like doing stomach crunches without realizing it!

Beauty Booster: Smiling makes you look younger and more attractive. Who doesn't want that?

Stress Relief: Recent research has shown that laughter significantly reduces your level of stress hormones like cortisol and adrenaline.

Improves Breathing: When you laugh, you inhale oxygen more deeply and empty air from your lungs more efficiently, which is especially good for anyone who suffers from respiratory conditions.

Lowers Blood Pressure: Laughing causes an increase in blood flow, which improves blood vessel function and lowers your blood pressure.

Protects against Heart Disease: By lowering your blood pressure, laughing helps to prevent heart disease. Taking in greater amounts of oxygen stimulates your heart and lungs.

Relieves Depression: When you laugh, your body releases feel-good endorphins as well as the mood-boosting hormone serotonin, which helps to reduce tension, make you less irritable, and put you in a better mood.

Improves Weight Loss: Laughing speeds up your metabolism, which increases the process of thermogenesis. This helps you burn more calories. In fact, 10 to 15 minutes of laughter each day can burn up to 50 calories, which translates into nearly 5 pounds of fat loss in a year!

Lowers Blood Sugar Levels. In one recent study, people living with diabetes attended a tedious lecture after eating a meal. The next day, the group ate the same meal and then watched a comedy. The group's blood sugar levels were lower after the funny film than the lecture.

Improves Sleep: Serotonin signals the brain to relax, which counters insomnia and sets the stage for better quality sleep.

Improves Memory: All that extra oxygen entering your bloodstream when you laugh fuels your brain, improving your ability to focus and boosting your memory.

Improves Social Life: Laughing easily and making other people laugh tends to improve your social relationships.

Boosts Creativity: Laughter's stress-relieving powers leave you feeling less preoccupied and better able to focus on creative tasks.

In sum, laughter is great for your overall health!

If you can't find anything to laugh about, SMILE. Studies show that a grin can help reduce symptoms associated with anxiety and can dramatically improve your mood. Do this simple test right now: Look straight ahead and smile as wide as you can. Now, try to think of something negative. It's hard, isn't it?

Smiling improves your odds of success, too. That's because people react more positively to you when you're perceived as upbeat, cheerful, and optimistic. They're more likely to go the extra mile to help you and to avoid picking a quarrel with you. In other words, wearing a more pleasant expression actually tends to make other people treat you more pleasantly. That paves the way to greater happiness for you and everyone you encounter. So, even when you feel insecure, blue, or frazzled, smile. You'll feel more confident and you'll get more positive results.

"You can't deny laughter; when it comes, it plops down in your favorite chair and stays as long as it wants."
—Stephen King

Beware Of Energy Vacuums!

We all know them. They're people who bring you down every time you're around them or talk to them on the phone. They leave you feeling drained and discouraged. Their energy is very negative.

Stop and think about the energy vacuums in your life. Make sure you surround yourself with upbeat people and limit your time with downers. Set boundaries. Spend more time with people who lift you up and leave you feeling inspired and positive and consciously spend less time with Negative Nellies. If you have to interact with energy vacuums, give yourself a pep talk afterward. Remind yourself that no one can ruin your day or drain your energy away, unless you let them.

If you can't think of any energy vacuums, you might just be one yourself! If so, it's time to replace pessimism and whining with optimism.

"The most wasted of all days is one without laughter."
—E.E. Cummings

Mental Nutrition®

Nourish your mind with positive information and always be open to personal development regardless of age. One of my favorite quotes from the late Jim Rohn, "The only thing worse than not reading a book in the last ninety days is not reading a book in the last ninety days and thinking that it doesn't matter". I want you to aim to read 10 pages a day of a book, preferably books that challenge you and help you to grow. Just by doing this, you will read over 15 books a year!

"Through humor, you can soften some of the worst blows that life delivers. And once you find laughter, no matter how painful your situation might be, you can survive it."
—Bill Cosby

---

10 Tips For Putting More Laughter Into Your Life

1. Pin funny sayings, pictures, and cartoons on your boards and look at them every day.
2. Find funny photos of yourself, your family, and your friends. Pin them. Add humorous captions, if you like.
3. Watch a classic comedy movie, a sitcom, or a silly cartoon.
4. Read humor books, comic strips, and humor websites.
5. Look in the mirror and make silly faces. Better yet, try making faces with your spouse or your child. Odds are, you'll both burst out laughing.
6. At dinner every evening, have each family member share one funny or embarrassing thing that happened that day.
7. Play with your pets and/or your kids. Enjoy their funny antics and facial expressions.
8. Try to find the funny side of seemingly serious situations. Next time you're angry, see if you can diffuse it with humor.
9. Include one light-hearted activity in every day. Even if you're not laughing while you're doing this, you're paving the way to a lighter-hearted, more laughter-filled life.
10. Include "find something humorous" in your daily To Do list. Don't cross it off until you've laughed aloud at least once.

"Laughter is the sun that drives winter from the human face."
—*Victor Hugo*

Sleep: The Pure Power Of A Good Night's Rest

Sleep is essential for a healthy body and mind, but most of us don't get nearly enough of it.

How much sleep do *you* need? Sleep requirements vary by individual and by age. Generally speaking, a one-year-old needs about 14 hours of shut-eye a night. A five-year-old needs about 12 hours of zzzzs. And an adult needs seven to eight hours a night. I'm talking about good, sound, uninterrupted sleep—not fitful tossing and turning.

Getting those hours of beauty rest every night can be a daunting task. But it's a must. Your body needs sleep for concentration, memory formation, repairing damaged cells, and reducing the risk of developing health problems like obesity, diabetes, and cardiovascular diseases.

What happens when you sleep? Your brain recharges and your body repairs itself. Getting adequate sleep helps you fight off infections and diseases. Even one sleepless night can lower your immune activity. Slumber also decreases your stress hormone production, your blood pressure, and the level of heart health-damaging inflammation in your body.

What's more, your brain processes information from the previous day more effectively when you're well-rested. Studies show that students who get a good night's sleep perform better on exams than those who cram all night. Why? Sleep deprivation makes it harder to concentrate, harder to think clearly, and harder to remember things. It slows down your reaction time and leaves you more prone to making mistakes, whether you're solving a math problem or operating heavy machinery. Not surprisingly, sleep deprivation increases your risk of being in a car accident.

"Laughter is an instant vacation."
—Milton Berle

5 Ways to Avoid Drowsy Driving

1. Try to get seven to eight hours of sleep EVERY night.
2. Whenever possible, adjust your schedule so that you're driving at times of the day when you're less likely to be drowsy.
3. Schedule regular breaks during long drives. Get out of the car, take deep breaths, and stretch to oxygenate your blood and clear your head.
4. If you're sleepy, find a safe rest area or parking lot where you can pull over and take a 15- to 20-minute nap.
5. Never drink ANY alcohol before you drive. Even if you're not over the legal limit, a glass of wine with dinner can make you a drowsy driver.
6. Whenever possible, avoid driving for long periods of time alone. If you've got another driver in the car with you, take turns at the wheel. Ask passengers to help you stay awake and to keep an eye on the traffic.

5 Reasons Sleep Matters

1. Safety. Skimping on sleep makes you more susceptible to errors and accidents on the job and behind the wheel.
2. Learning. Sleep is essential to your brain's ability to transfer new information to memory.
3. Heart health. Poor sleep habits contribute to hypertension and increased stress hormone levels, which sets the stage for heart attacks, strokes, and cardiovascular disease.
4. Immune function. Sleep deprivation can lower your immune system and make you more apt to get sick. Some studies also suggest that sleep helps the body fight cancer.
5. Mood. When you don't get enough sleep, you're more likely to be cranky, short-tempered, and generally no fun to be around.

Zzzzs: The Key Ingredient To Successful Weight Loss?

Can you lose weight while you snooze? It sounds like a dream, but getting adequate sleep each night can actually help to control your body weight. That's because sleep helps to regulate the hormones that affect appetite. As you know now, ghrelin stimulates your appetite, while leptin sends a signal to your brain that you've eaten enough. People who don't get enough sleep have lower leptin levels and higher ghrelin levels—and that can lead to overeating.

Studies show that when you sleep seven to eight hours a night, you eat about 300 calories less than when you only sleep about four hours. Plus, when you're sleep-deprived and your appetite spikes, you tend to crave comfort foods high in sugar and fat. And to make matters even worse, when you're short on sleep, your body constantly produces the stress hormone cortisol, which can trigger all kinds of problems, including:

- Inflammation
- Insomnia
- Fat storage and weight gain (I know you DON'T want this!)
- Reduced growth hormone production
- Decreased immunity
- Decreased short-term memory
- Decreased muscle tone

"The secret of health for both mind and body is not to mourn for the past, worry about the future, but to live in the present moment wisely and earnestly." —Buddha

9 Tips For A Good Night's Rest

Try these simple tips to help you drift off peacefully and wake up refreshed and ready to tackle the day.

1. **Be consistent.** Try to go to sleep and get up at the same time every day, even on the weekends and on vacation.

2. **Don't snack.** Never eat or drink before bedtime, especially caffeinated beverages. (Remember: no eating after 7:30 p.m. on *The Pinterest Diet!*)

3. **Calm down.** Create a soothing nightly bedtime routine for yourself. Take a bubble bath, listen to calming music, light a candle and meditate. Borrow a trick that parents of newborns use: Lower the lights and sound in your home an hour before bedtime. This signals your brain that you're winding down for the night and triggers your body to start producing melatonin, which helps you sleep.

   Resist the urge to check your Twitter and email accounts before bed. Researchers have found that people who shut down their phones, TV, and laptops at least an hour before bedtime get a better night's rest.

4. **Curb stress.** Keep anxiety triggers out of your bedroom. Don't stack work or newspapers on your nightstand. Never leave your laptop next to your bed. Every time you see them, your brain automatically gets more alert. Your blood pressure might even spike and your heart rate might increase. Even the most fleeting thoughts about your endless To Do list or the massive client project you'll never finish by the deadline can sabotage your ability to sleep. So can a glimpse of the latest headlines about wars, crimes, or layoffs.

   If you can't bear to leave your cell phone in the living room, turn it off and tuck it in the top drawer of your dresser (unless you're using it for the sound machine app below).

   Finally, never fight at night. Save stressful conversations with family members and friends for the next day.

5. **Rig the room.** Make sure your bedroom is cool, dark, and quiet when you're trying to sleep. Invest in blackout shades, earplugs, and an eye mask. (I've tried many over the years, and my favorite is a simple $3 model from the pharmacy section of Walmart.)

   Buy a white noise machine or download a sound machine app on your smartphone. The one I use is Sleep Machine for iPhone. It cost me

$1.99, and it was well worth the investment because I use it every night and always have it with me when I travel. You might also consider playing soothing music to help yourself fall asleep.

What's the ideal temperature for the bedroom? Most people sleep best when the room is between 68 and 72 degrees.

Did you know? According to one recent survey, 35% of smartphone users would choose their phones over their spouses! And 87% bring their phones into their bedroom.

"Work for a cause, not for applause. Live life to express, not to impress. Don't strive to let your presence noticed, just make your absence felt."
—Anonymous

6. **Set the stage.** Invest in a comfortable bed, bedding, and pillows. Don't skimp on the pillows! My favorites are Tempur-Pedic. Generally speaking, thinner, flatter pillows work better if you sleep on your back or stomach. Side sleepers need firmer, plumper pillows to prevent aching necks and shoulders. (If you suffer from back pain, you might also want to tuck a small pillow between your knees to keep your hips and spine aligned when you lie on your side.) Whatever type of pillows you choose, experts recommend replacing them every 12 to 18 months.

   Also, investing in some high-quality sheets has helped me get a better night's sleep. I buy mine on Overstock.com. They're on my Mitzi's Favorite Products Board. Love them!

   If you've got allergies, purchase zippered hypoallergenic cases for your mattress and pillows to avoid lying awake suffering from a runny nose, sneezing, and wheezing. If your pet is triggering your allergies, talk to your vet about retraining him or her to sleep in his own bed at the foot of yours or in another room altogether.

7. **Stay away during the day.** Your bed should be used exclusively for sleep and sex—never for work, chatting on the phone, or paying bills. That way your brain begins to associate your bed with relaxation. Even

walking into your bedroom cues your subconscious mind that it's time to sleep.

8. **Unplug it.** Studies show that the blue light emitted by electronic devices like cell phones, TVs, and digital clocks can short-circuit your sleep. Put your alarm clock in a drawer, under the bed, or turn it around so you can't see it.

9. **Get done earlier.** Make a schedule for yourself and complete important tasks—especially those that require intense concentration and that raise your anxiety level—earlier in the day, so you have time to relax before bed.

The same holds true for working out. Research shows that regular exercise helps you sleep better, but not if you do it right before bedtime. If you're struggling with insomnia, check out the National Sleep Foundation's website, at SleepFoundation.org

"Sleep is the best meditation."
—Dalai Lama

Stress Management: Unwinding Can
Help You Live A Longer, Better Life

Whether it's the pressures of work, family, or daily life, stress comes at us from all angles. And it can be truly debilitating. It can endanger your health and lead you to destructive coping mechanisms, from smoking to popping prescription tranquilizers. Its side effects run the gamut from headaches, insomnia, and jaw pain (TMJ) to weight gain, depression, and heart disease.

We know stress is a killer, but we can't seem to escape it. Based on one recent large-scale survey by the American Psychological Association, nearly half of all Americans are worried about the level of stress in their lives. And 65% of us are losing sleep due to stress, according to additional data.

No one wants to live a life riddled with anxiety. The good news is you don't have to! The best way to combat the stress in your life is to develop a strategy that helps you cope with the specific issues and times that tend to make you feel overwhelmed by life's pressures. When do you feel most stressed? On Sunday nights, with a week's worth of work looming ahead? When a birthday approaches and you start cataloguing all the things you didn't accomplish this year? When the kids start bickering? When your mom calls? Once you've identified the major stressors in your life, you can develop some coping strategies.

As always, Pinterest is a great place to start. It's a terrific source of stress management advice, tips, and information. It's replete with boards of inspiring quotes, healthy recipes, workouts, and DIY de-stressing projects. Collect the ones that speak to you.

Here are some of my favorite Pinterest-approved stress busters.

1. **Sweat it out.** When you exercise, your body releases endorphins, which instantly boost your mood. A good workout will keep you in shape, give you a sense of accomplishment, and leave you feeling better about your body. It will also quell the negative effects of stress on your body. Check out my Workout Plans Board for a variety of stress-relieving workouts.

2. **Eat well.** It's tempting to reach for the nearest bag of potato chips and start crunching away your tension. But that's the worst thing you can do. You'll end up feeling sluggish, bloated, and guilty—all of which will make you stressed out all over again. (And the number on the bathroom scale won't help!) Instead, choose foods rich in disease-fighting antioxidants, fiber, protein, and healthy fats. MSF Factor Foods such as avocados and salmon will give you staying power. (For more great food choices, check out the list of six super choices below.) By eating a variety of nutrient-rich foods, you'll avoid blood sugar spikes and maintain normal glucose levels, all of which make it easier to manage your stress.

3. **Make time for yourself.** Take a break from the daily grind, even if it's just for ten minutes a day. Use your mini-break to decompress and pamper yourself. Push stressful thoughts to the back of your mind. Turn off your cell phone. Find a quiet spot and ask your family not to bother you for 10 minutes. Try a DIY Pinterest beauty project like a hair mask, a facial, aromatherapy with essential oils, meditation, or yoga. Use the time to recharge your batteries—to fill yourself with renewed energy and motivation. (By the way, this time should be in addition to your daily 10 minutes of pinning.)

> *"A well-spent day brings happy sleep."*
> *—Leonardo da Vinci*

Mitzi's Super Six

The breathlessly fast-paced lifestyle has become ingrained in American culture. We've become ultra-productive multi-tasking masters, but our never-ending sprint has triggered a significant rise in stress-related illness in the U.S. Here's why: Stress increases the body's production of free radicals, which can wreak havoc on your health. The six foods below contain compounds that fight back against dangerous free radicals. Eat them often to help your body balance the damaging effect of daily stress.

1. **Almonds** contain vitamin B2 and vitamin E, which limit production of harmful free radicals.
2. **Spinach** contains the mineral magnesium. Magnesium is responsible for the production of GABA, which helps your body produce the neuro-transmitter dopamine, connected with pleasure.
3. **Strawberries** are packed with vitamin C, which also combats free radical production.
4. **Sweet potatoes** satisfy cravings for sweets and carbs without overloading your body with sugar. Sweet potatoes also contain health-promoting beta-carotene and other vitamins.
5. **Turkey** contains the amino acid L-tryptophan, which activates the release of serotonin, a mood-boosting neurotransmitter.
6. **Asparagus** is packed with folic acid, which helps your body manufacture dopamine.

Mitzi's Picks

Check out UP by Jawbone. You can find this handy bracelet-style health and fitness tool at Apple stores and online for $129.99. I love mine. It tells me how many steps I've taken each day and—my favorite feature—how many hours of deep sleep and light sleep I got the night before. It even keeps track of how many times I woke up! Analyzing this information helps me figure out ways to improve my sleep habits and, ultimately, get a better night's sleep.

"The greatest weapon against stress is our
ability to choose one thought over another."
—William James

Need more stress reducers? Try these.

- **Talk through it.** If you can find a sympathetic ear—whether it's a spouse, a friend, or a therapist—discussing stressful situations can be cathartic. Just make sure you're not increasing the listener's stress level in the process!

> *"There's going to be stress in life, but it's your*
> *choice whether to let it affect you or not."*
> *—Valerie Bertinelli*

- **Re-assess stress.** Feeling helpless aggravates stress. Remind yourself that you have more control of your life and decisions than you might think. If you're feeling overwhelmed, are you procrastinating? Being a perfectionist? Avoiding prioritizing? Could you delegate some tasks to other people? Recognizing the part you play in creating or maintaining stress in your life is the first step toward making changes for the better.
- Identify the main sources of stress in your life and start trying to find ways to reduce them or eliminate them altogether. If you can't remove the stressors, can you change the way you react to them? Could you compromise, lower your standards, or say "no" more often?
- **Volunteer.** Studies show that helping other people can reduce stress.
- **Connect with others.** Spending time with people you enjoy is a great way to decompress and unwind. It alleviates the sense of isolation and makes you feel loved and supported emotionally. Scientists have found that people who have strong social connections and close relationships with others are happier and healthier.
- **Have fun.** Make time for leisure activities that make you happy.
- **Reprogram your thoughts.** Negative self-talk leaves you feeling defeated before you start. Next time you catch yourself thinking, "I'll never get everything done" or "I can't cope," STOP. Take a deep breath. Tell yourself, "Yes, I can. I CAN cope. I can get the things that matter most done." Even an

internal message as simple as "My best IS good enough" can do wonders for your outlook and your self-esteem.

- Need a few more inspirational sayings? Time to visit your Daily Inspiration Board on Pinterest—or mine!

Pinterest Pointer: Remember to consult my In The Know Board for tips, tricks, and tools to help you get a better night's rest.

A Mitzi Moment: Discussing Stress with Dr. Oz

I was recently invited to be a guest on *The Dr. Oz Show* to talk about foods that help to reduce stress. I got the call on a Sunday during a holiday weekend when I was out of town at a volleyball tournament in a crowded convention center. With more than 50 volleyball courts and whistles blowing constantly, the noise was deafening. I didn't get home until late Monday night, and my flight to New York City left the next day! The *Dr. Oz Show* taping was scheduled for Wednesday.

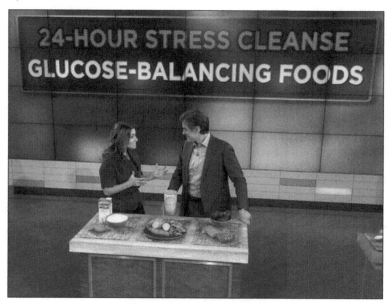

On The Dr. Oz Show

"Train like an athlete, eat like a nutritionist,
sleep like a baby, win like a champion."
—*Anonymous*

I've appeared on television more than 300 times during my career, but this time was different. I'd spoken in front of live audiences a few times, but never any as prominent as Dr. Oz's.

In the very first segment of the show, another physician was talking to Dr. Oz about how to breathe to help reduce your heart rate when you're stressed. I was so stressed that I felt like my heart was going to pop out of my chest. I was literally practicing what she was saying about breathing. I was in segment two and, as soon as he had finished talking with her, Dr. Oz walked over to me.

Once my segment started, I calmed down and the segment was great fun, but I'll never forget my first appearance on *The Dr. Oz Show,* when discussing stress-reducing foods caused me to have three of the most stressed-out days of my life. Ha!

"Inhale the best, exhale the stress."
—*Anonymous*

Conquering Your Cortisol Levels To Lose Fat

Here's another incentive to calm down! The stress hormone cortisol, secreted by your adrenal gland, can sabotage your weight loss efforts.

First, it can lead to more fat storage (specifically in the abdomen . . . which I KNOW you don't want).

Second, it can increase your appetite and your cravings for high-calorie foods.

When you're anxious, frazzled, and short on sleep, your cortisol levels spike. With time, those unhealthy elevated cortisol levels can wreak havoc on your health.

"Dear stress. Let's break up."
—*Anonymous*

More Healthy Living Hints

In addition to laughing often, sleeping enough, and lowering your stress level, here are a few tips to help you take better care of yourself.

1. **Read a positive-thinking book.** Two of my favorite authors are Jack Canfield, success coach and co-creator of the Chicken Soup series, and leadership expert John Maxwell.
2. **Surround yourself with positive, upbeat people.**
3. **Keep setbacks and frustrations in perspective.** As author Richard Carlson put it, "Don't sweat the small stuff—and it's all small stuff."
4. **Let go of your worries before you go to bed each night.**
5. **Be present each day for life and love.** In other words, live in the moment. Don't be so preoccupied by your phone that you ignore your family and friends who are with you. Enjoy life as it happens instead of worrying about the future or dwelling on the past.

"Never let the things you want make you
forget the things you have."
—*Anonymous*

CHAPTER 13:

THE PINTEREST DIET ON A BUDGET

Think you've got to shell out more money to eat healthier? Not necessarily. There are lots of ways to whittle down your grocery bill as you whittle down your waist. Try these 20 strategies to get better nutrition without breaking the bank.

1. Make a plan and stick to it. Set aside 30 minutes every Sunday to plan your week's menus. Log onto Pinterest and find at least two new recipes to make in the next seven days. Then fill out a weekly meal chart that includes breakfast, lunch, dinner, and a daily optional snack. As you plan, think about your schedule for the week. Are parent-teacher conferences coming up? Will you be working late to meet a looming deadline? If you're anticipating a hectic schedule, choose meals that are quick and easy to make.

Make a list of the ingredients you'll need for each meal. Be sure you check your pantry to find out what you already have. Add any items you'll need to buy to your list. Buy ONLY what's on your list. You'll avoid unnecessary purchases and you won't be tempted to splurge on overpriced food deliveries or take-out dinners.

Raid Your Cupboards!

Before you finalize your menus for the week and make a grocery list, check your own pantry, refrigerator, and freezer to find out what foods you have on hand. Have you tucked away a container of breadcrumbs and canned tomatoes? If so, why not pick up some fresh eggplant and make a delicious eggplant Parmesan? If you've got brown rice and a jar of salsa, why not pick up some fresh peppers and onions and whip up a zesty vegetarian Mexican rice dish? Finding creative ways to use the ingredients you have at home is a great way to save money at the grocery store.

---

2. Make foods do double duty. If you'll need tomatoes for one meal, choose a second meal that includes tomatoes. If you're baking a chicken, use the leftovers for a salad or sandwich the next day for lunch. Or sprinkle some shredded chicken on top of black beans for a savory, protein-filled lunch. This trick not only saves money, but it makes meal prep much easier. You can also make double batches of MSF Factor Foods casseroles, chili, soups, and stews and freeze them for future meals on nights when you're too tired to cook anything from scratch.

3. Know when organic is worth the price. I always recommend organic 1% milk and organic apples, but generally speaking, fruits and veggies with thick, removable skins don't have to be organic. These include bananas, melons, pineapple, and eggplant. Caveat: Always wash your produce well with water to get as much of the pesticides off as possible.

4. Eat smaller portions of meat. Instead of making meat the star of your meals, make it a team player by including it but shifting the focus to other ingredients. If you're creative, you can stretch small portions of pork tenderloin or chicken breast into two family meals with the addition of whole grains and lots of veggies. A family of four can share two steaks when the meat is sliced up for kebabs or stir-fry. Cuts like sirloin, round eye, lean ground beef, and flank are leaner and less expensive than New York Strip and just as delicious. Tenderize cheaper cuts with a meat mallet or marinade. (Check out my Pinterest boards for mouthwatering marinade recipes!)

5. Eat greens to save green. Include a few vegetarian meals in your weekly menu. Eat protein-rich plant-based foods like beans (black, garbanzo, kidney, etc.), lentils, and quinoa. They're nutritious, delicious, versatile, and cheap. Add them to salads, pasta, soups, and more. You can also buy eggs, onions, baby carrots, and celery for pennies per serving. They're nutritious and easy to add to lots of different dishes.

6. Buy store brands. House brands of foods like brown rice, whole wheat pasta, canned beans, and frozen vegetables are just as tasty as costlier name brands. One great example of this is Walmart's Great Value product line. In 2011, Walmart committed to making food healthier, affordable, and accessible, setting a goal to reformulate thousands of their Great Value items by 2015. They've already made great strides in lowering sodium, sugar, and trans fats. As a part of the program, they wanted to help customers easily identify healthier choices, so they developed a "Great For You" icon as a simple front-of-package seal.

7. Buy in season. Produce is at its freshest and cheapest when it's in season because it's plentiful and doesn't have to be shipped far. Find out what's in season in your region, and plan your meals accordingly. If you're not sure, check out my In The Know Board for seasonal produce tips. Why not create a Pinterest board of seasonal recipes to make sure you have the freshest, most satisfying and affordable meals at your fingertips?

8. Never shop when you're hungry. You know what happens when you do: You fill your grocery cart up with spur-of-the-moment items . . . and they're usually not the smartest, healthiest ones.

9. Invest in the right appliances. If you're on a tight budget, choose one or two multi-tasking appliances you can use to prepare wholesome meals. I recommend a George Foreman Grill because it grills everything from lean burgers and chicken to Paninis—all of which are easy and healthful ways to prepare your meals. A high-quality blender is an ideal investment too. I love mine. I use it to make smoothies at least once a day.

10. Bulk up. Buy items like beans, oatmeal, whole wheat pasta, brown rice, rolled oats, frozen fruits, and frozen vegetables in bulk from wholesale warehouses. If you don't have room to store bulkier items, portion them into smaller clear or clearly labeled food storage containers. Caveat: The only items you should buy in bulk are the ones you eat often and enjoy, and that fit into *The Pinterest Diet.* Don't buy foods in bulk that will tempt you and challenge your willpower!

11. Track your calories. Keeping track of your calories in a journal or through an app will not only help you manage your weight and your food intake, it will also help you avoid spending on extras that are bad for both your waistline and your wallet.

12. Stock up on frozen vegetables. Eat veggies at every meal. Include fresh ones whenever possible, but don't be afraid to supplement with frozen versions. They're often picked at the peak of their ripeness and flash frozen immediately to lock in their nutrients. Instead of letting fruits or veggies spoil in the fridge, you can freeze them yourself. I love doing this with ripe bananas.

13. Check the top and bottom shelves. Some grocery stores tend to tuck the lower-priced items away from eye-level.

14. Do the prep work yourself. Sure, foods that have been peeled, chopped, cooked, or otherwise assembled for you are convenient, but convenience adds cost. Slice and dice yourself. You'll slice your food budget in the process.

Freeze It!

In addition to fruits and veggies, you can freeze meat, bread, butter, herbs, mashed avocado, and even eggs cracked open and stored in an airtight container. For information on how to freeze specific foods, try these websites:

- OrganicGardening.com/cook/freezing-basics
- NCHFP.uga.edu/how/freeze.html.

---

15. Clip coupons. It's an old strategy, but a good one. Plan your dinners around what's healthy and on sale. Check the Sunday supplements of your local newspaper and read the posters in the grocery store windows advertising the latest deals.

16. Shop at a lower-cost grocery store. Many lower-cost grocery stores offer lots of healthy options. Save more expensive neighborhood grocery stores for last-minute emergency trips.

17. Get creative in the kitchen. Craving pizza but don't want to fork over the money to get it delivered? Keep a jar of pizza sauce in the cupboards and some low-fat mozzarella in your refrigerator. Instead of premade pizza dough, use whole wheat sandwich thins or tortillas. Use your imagination to find tasty new dishes featuring inexpensive ingredients.

18. Eat out less often. Restaurants are pricey—not to mention fattening. You save money and have more control of what goes into your meals when you dine in. If you're a parent, it's wise to teach your children to cook at an early age. Besides, the kitchen is a great place to create good family memories.

19. Be smart when you eat out. Don't blow your budget calorie-wise or dollar-wise by ordering alcohol and dessert. Choose one or the other. Or neither. Another great way to curb costs and calories is to order an appetizer instead of an entrée (the portions are often huge) as your main course or share an entrée with a friend or family member.

20. Grow your own. Whether it's a small organic herb garden with basil, chives, and rosemary or a big vegetable garden with tomatoes, kale, and carrots, growing your own food can help you keep grocery bills in check. It's also a great family project if you've got kids.

BONUS TIP: Shop at farmers' markets. Go when the market is about to close; that's when farmers tend to slash produce prices. Also, find the biggest markets. With more vendors, there's more competition, which means better prices. Visit LocalHarvest.org to find a market near your home.

CHAPTER 14:

SATISFIED FOREVER

"Our greatest weakness lies in giving up. The most certain way to succeed is always to try one more time."
—*Thomas Edison*

They say every journey comes to an end. But the journey doesn't *really* end here. You'll continue to make amazing progress, using the simple, sensible principles you've learned in this book. Soon you'll reach your health, weight loss, and fitness goals.

Achieving those goals will open the door to a whole new level of fulfillment and happiness in your life. You'll have more energy to do the things you love. You'll have more confidence and courage to try the things you've always wanted to do. And you'll be filled with newfound optimism because you'll know you can succeed. You'll appreciate how unlimited your potential really is because you've blasted through old roadblocks, overcome challenges, and accomplished results you thought were unattainable. You've discovered strength you never knew you possessed.

Talk about life transformation!

Even after you reach your weight loss goals, keep this book handy and keep pinning for at least 10 minutes *every day*. You know as well as I do by now that Pinterest

> ### Pinterest Tip: Remember To "Pin 10" With Time Blocking
>
> This technique helps me tremendously when I need to get anything done more efficiently. Log off your email account and turn off your cell phone ringer. Use your smartphone only as your 10-minute timer (unless you're pinning from your cell phone). You can also use an old-fashioned kitchen timer, a wristwatch timer, or an online or computer timer. Don't check messages, answer calls, or let anything else distract you until the timer goes off. Immerse yourself fully in Pinterest for this block of time. Enjoy!

is an endless, ever-changing treasure trove brimming with creative ideas and inspirational photos. Whenever there's a new health breakthrough, a hot fashion trend, or an innovative twist on working out, check my boards and other reliable resources on Pinterest for tips on how to apply it to your own life. Also, refer to my boards, your boards, and this book whenever you need a refresher.

> *"Good things come to those who work*
> *their asses off and never give up."*
> —*Anonymous*

Share Your Successes With Me

I love hearing from you! Getting your emails and Facebook posts is the very best part of my work. I read everything you write to me. So let me know what you liked most about *The Pinterest Diet*. What items on my boards did you find most helpful? What else would you like to see me pinning? What were the biggest challenges you faced? Share your stories with me, and I'll share them on my Success Stories Board. (Don't worry; I'll always ask your permission before I post them!)

Here's How To Connect With Me:

Facebook: Facebook.com/NutritionExpert
Instagram: Instagram.com/NutritionExpert
LinkedIn: LinkedIn.com/in/MitziDulan
Pinterest: Pinterest.com/NutritionExpert
Twitter: Twitter.com/NutritionExpert
YouTube: YouTube.com/TheNutritionExpert

Pin My Book!

If you enjoyed *The Pinterest Diet*, please share it on your Pinterest boards. You can visit my website, NutritionExpert.com, for book images or pin the book cover directly from Amazon.com.

Rewards For You!

As my way of saying thanks for buying my book and taking this 30-day journey toward better health and fitness with me, I'd like to offer you **FOUR FREE** Pinterest Diet Party Gifts, available exclusively for my readers:

- A bonus book chapter available as an e-book! Chapter 15: Pin Your Way Thin In 10 Minutes A Day provides a Sunday-to-Saturday daily pinning plan.
- *The Pinterest Diet* Shopping List: Your Guide to Navigating the Grocery Store makes combing the aisles for healthy, nutrient-rich items a cinch.
- *The Pinterest Diet* Goal Sheet: to allow you to write down your goals, reread daily, and take action.
- *The Pinterest Diet* Food Log: write down your food intake onto this sheet to keep track of what you are eating. You will be more successful if you follow this one simple step.

"The difference between the possible and impossible lies in the person's determination."
—Anonymous

To claim your gifts, just visit my website at NutritionExpert.com. All are available as downloadable PDF files. They're terrific supplements to the information provided in *The Pinterest Diet*.

Get Free News Updates From Me!

The best way to keep up on the latest Pinterest Diet news is to sign up for my e-newsletter. I'll keep you up to date on my latest blog posts, important links, new videos, and I'll announce any Pinterest Parties, Twitter Parties or Pinterest Contests this way as well. Just go to NutritionExpert.com and click on the purple button in the red bar at the top to register for free.

BONUS GIFT! When you sign up for my e-newsletter, I'll give you a complimentary copy of my e-book *56 Simple Ways to Lose Weight Without Dieting*.

Final Thoughts . . .

Small Steps Lead To Big Results!

We all get discouraged from time to time. And it's easy to let a "bad" day stretch into a bad week or even a bad month. Before you know it, you give up. Soon it's next year and there you are AGAIN making ANOTHER New Year's Resolution to lose weight.

I want to make sure that never happens to you again. Remember, *it's okay to fall off the wagon* once in a while. The key to genuine life transformation is getting up, dusting yourself off, and climbing back *on* the healthy-living wagon! Never beat yourself up when you make a mistake. Be as forgiving of yourself as would be of someone you love. Reprogram those self-defeating, browbeating internal messages with encouraging ones. *Don't give up. You can do it. Just get back on track.*

No one eats perfectly all the time. That's okay. Strive for small, consistent improvements. Eventually, they'll give you big results.

Eat Real. Move Often. Laugh Much. Live Fully.

ABOUT THE AUTHOR

Mitzi Dulan, RD, America's Nutrition Expert®, is one of the most highly recognized nutritionists in the country. She's an-award winning, internationally known, registered dietitian, speaker, nutrition spokesperson, author, and certified personal trainer, who has inspired millions to lose weight and get fit. With her unique blend of high energy and down-to-earth charm, Mitzi passionately motivates people to take action. Mitzi is the co-author of *The All-Pro Diet* with NFL future Hall-of-Famer Tony Gonzalez, helping people eat clean and get lean.

She is the team nutritionist for the Kansas City Royals Baseball Team. She has also previously served as the longtime team nutritionist for the Kansas City Chiefs Football Team.

Mitzi is a sought-after media source for trusted nutrition and fitness information. She has conducted more than 300 television interviews across the country and has been a featured guest on *The Dr. Oz Show* and CNN. She appears regularly on FOX News Channel and is a blogger for *U.S. News & World Report*.

Mitzi is frequently quoted in publications, such as *The Wall Street Journal, Newsweek, US Weekly, Family Circle, USA Today, Men's Fitness, Maxim, Glamour, Women's World, Fitness, Oxygen, Prevention, First,* the *San Francisco Chronicle,* and the *San Jose Mercury News* as well as online at HuffingtonPost.com, ESPN.com, MSN.com, FoodNetwork.com, Forbes.com, AOL.com, Yahoo.com, Shape.com, and Glamour.com. She has been a speaker for a number of Fortune 500 companies as well as for the U.S. Army and Morgan Stanley.

Mitzi has developed a highly engaged social media following on all of her social media outlets. She has more than three million followers on Pinterest and was named one of the Top 20 Nutrition Experts to Follow on Twitter by The Huffington Post. She was also named the #5 online influencer to help Americans Eat Better by ShareCare.com, behind Dr. Weil and Jamie Oliver.

Mitzi earned her dual B.S. degrees in Nutrition and Exercise Science, graduating cum laude in both from Kansas State University. She burst onto the nutrition scene and was awarded Recognized Young Dietitian of the Year by the Academy of Nutrition and Dietetics and won Kansas State University's *Entrepreneur of the Year* award.

When not traveling to share her message of persistence and hard work, you will find her at home living the lifestyle she teaches with her husband and two daughters. She loves experimenting with new recipes and cooking clean, real foods that are full of flavor. She lives in Kansas City.

To learn more about Mitzi and to find her latest recipes, visit NutritionExpert. com and follow her on Pinterest at Pinterest.com/NutritionExpert.

Work With Me!

If you own or work with a food, fitness, or health company or commodity board and feel that your products would be a good fit with my brand of clean eating, fitness, and healthy living, please contact my manager, Julie May at Julie@MediaMotionIntl.com I provide social media services, book signings, and traditional media and speaking engagements.

INDEX

CPSIA information can be obtained at www.ICGtesting.com
Printed in the USA
LVOW01s0015010214

371745LV00008B/267/P

9 780989 723947